Creating Peace with Your Hands

Prevention and Self-Care for the Manual Therapist

Karina Braun, BAAS, LMT

Creating Peace with Your Hands

Cover art by Karina Braun

ISBN:
978-0-9816199-0-3

Library of Congress Control Number:
2008911240

Please visit website at
www.igetintouch.com

Get In Touch Publishing
5546 Camino Al Norte #2-173
N. Las Vegas, NV 89031

Printed in the USA
By Morris Publishing
3212 East Highway 30
Kearney, NE 68847
800-650-7888

Preface

This book contains information to assist manual therapists. This book is for any manual therapist, including massage therapist, bodyworker, or one that has a hand intensive occupation. Most of the terminology in this book will consist of therapist, massage therapist, and bodyworker, but it could apply to any manual therapist or one that uses his/her hands repetitively in their career. Strategies, ideas, and exercises will be presented to prolong your career. This book will enhance your understanding of working smart, not hard.

<u>Dedication</u>

This book is dedicated to all of you who take pride in helping others. This earth and the people on it need some serious healing for positive change to happen. With your help, we can heal the world one person at a time.

Acknowledgements

I am thankful for many wonderful people that assisted me in so many ways while I wrote this book. The universe supported me in writing this book even if it came in a way I might not have expected. I am grateful for:

My Mom for her constant love, support, and editing skills.

Krista for her love and knowledge of yoga.

My Dad, Kathy, Kenton, and Keiran for their love, support, and honest opinions.

My great friend Janene for her support, feedback, and photography skills.

Cy for her editing, friendship, and creativity.

All of my friends for the extra support including, but not limited to: Ellen, Sigi, Tertia, Steve, Lee Beam, Kim, Mary, Sue, Meagan, and Angel.

Veronica for her great editing skills.

Dr. Borgia, Adell, Dr. Nicola, Cleo, David Teper, Deb Lazarski, Dr. Flaviano, and Dr. Kelley for their support, treatment, and assistance in my healing.

I want to thank each and every client along the way because without you I would not have had the knowledge to write this book.

Finally, thank you Jeff for your love, encouragement, and belief in me. You helped me with my healing and gave me the support I needed to finish this book.

Foreword

The profession of massage and bodywork has become big business and has evolved into a major industry in the last decade. Massage therapy is currently more accepted as a therapeutic modality than in the past. This demand for treatment has created more full-time work for massage therapists and higher expectations have been placed on schools to train more qualified therapists. These factors have added more pressure and have increased chances of injury to the performing therapists.

Today, the industry faces many challenges. Schools are not taking the time to train each student on how to use his/her body properly or how to use the equipment ergonomically. The demand for massage is greater but the techniques have gotten deeper and more intricate. Injury prevention is complex and it needs to be understood completely for bodyworkers to steer clear of any injuries. Therapists must first understand what their physical advantages and limitations are and learn how to use their body correctly. Bodyworkers must understand how to care for their body before, during, and after performing a massage.

Schools and working facilities must emphasize body mechanics and self-care combined together. Some clinics and spas look more at the profit in money than the protection of their own therapists' interests. A lot of times, therapists are not allowed more than five minutes between appointments, they work eight to ten hour shifts, and they hardly have room to move around the table. These facilities must not have the mentality of thinking that each therapist is a number. They must maintain an attitude of taking each person and their attributes and limitations into consideration.

On the other hand, therapists think of themselves as caregivers and believe it is not acceptable to be injured because they have the tendency to put others needs before their own. I believe that bodyworkers do not have a full understanding of the physiology of injury and also have shame when they are injured. Occupational injuries are very high in this field. If the statistics are to improve, bodyworkers need to stand up and voice what is going on with them so that other therapists will feel more comfortable to do so. Shame will only make having an injury worse. If you say nothing and work through your injury, you could make the situation worse. Fear is a common emotion when you have symptoms of an injury because you may be fearful of losing your income or your job. It is a shame that you have to be afraid when it comes to using your body for your work. Priorities need to be set so that your body's needs are being put first. You have to have awareness of your own body and stop doing an activity when certain symptoms arise in order to avoid becoming your own worst enemy.

The massage field has come a long way in the last decade. It will be a positive step in the right direction if schools teach injury prevention as a foundation. Therapists need to think holistically by doing full-body massage instead of only performing spot work. Bodyworkers need to step up and not be afraid to speak of their injury in hopes of helping others.

In addition to thinking about injury prevention and your health for the present moment, you also need to think about staying healthy for the long-term. Even with good body mechanics, ergonomics, and self-care an injury can happen. It is important to prepare yourself for the future by incorporating new modalities and techniques that are easier on your body. Smart and healthy choices today will ensure a safe and healthy career for tomorrow.

Table of Contents

Introduction

From an early age, I knew I had a healing touch and felt like I was here on earth to assist people through touch. I always had a lot of enthusiasm and needed an outlet for my energy. In high school I enjoyed putting my energy into playing sports but I still needed more creativity in my life. I always knew I needed a career that was physical as well as inspiring. I attended the University of North Texas and studied psychology, sociology, and criminal justice. I took a philosophy class my senior year of college and got to know myself better. This inspiring class helped me to understand more about life itself.

At this time, my mother was in pain and recovering from back surgery. I was on a mission to find an alternative therapy that would reduce her pain and help her to heal. Massage therapy was the approach that helped relieve my mom's muscle contractions and lessen her pain. Through this process, I found out that I wanted to go into a career in the healing arts because I could help people and I could work for myself, independently. I explored many of the healing arts and soon figured out that massage therapy would be my career after college. In 1997, after graduating college I enrolled in massage school in Dallas and after 300 hours of training, I was prepared with great knowledge and touch in Swedish massage. My instructors were wonderful in their teachings of anatomy, physiology, and technique, but the subject of using my own body mechanics to do massage was minimal.

After completing my massage internship, I got married and started my own business. I could not wait to show the passion and creativity I had for my art. I bought a salon along with a hairdresser and prepared the back room as a comfortable and tranquil massage space. I assisted in the remodeling of the salon and, during that process, I strained my lower back. I was not thinking of my body during this time because I was excited about the future and ready to get started. I did not allow time for myself to exercise or to stretch. After getting my massage business up and running, I aggravated my low back further because I was performing deep tissue massage incorrectly on my clients. I was twisting my low back while I was applying pressure. My clients were getting the correct results but I was in pain. Here I was only twenty-three years old, at the beginning of my career, in pain, and wondering where to turn for help. From that day on, I would read and absorb everything I could get my hands on to help me understand low back mechanisms and body mechanics. Finding information on body mechanics for bodyworkers was challenging ten years ago; however, I learned whatever I could with the small amount of information that I gathered. The upside of experiencing this injury was that I had an increased understanding of my clients' low back pain and the many difficulties that are associated with it.

It was time to implement some self-care and body awareness to my routine. I attended Tai Chi classes for six weeks to gain body awareness and movement. I started to do warm-up stretches at the start of my day and then in between each massage. I found that consistent stretching kept my low back from hurting. My search for answers led me to yoga and enhanced my massage treatments. Practicing yoga lessened my pain and made me more patient, flexible, and grounded. In addition to practicing yoga, I entered the kickboxing scene. Kickboxing helped me to strengthen my low back and hip muscles because I did a lot of abdominal exercises, plyometrics, and kicking drills. The moderate punching helped condition the tendons in my arms and the cardiovascular exercise sent more oxygen to my muscles, giving me more energy to do my work. My back finally healed about six months after the injury because I was proactive and took the time to care for my body.

Awareness of my own body, along with strengthening and stretching became a part of my daily routine. I knew if I ignored these parts of my routine, my back would hurt. I was sure that yoga had been my main teacher and so my next step was to study and become a certified yoga teacher. I studied a blend of Viniyoga, Ashtanga, and Iyengar yoga and challenged myself in every facet of my studies. I received my yoga teacher certification in 2001. I was now not only able to offer massage to my clients, but was also able to share the concept of self-care by teaching them yoga.

Living with a musician, at the time, was both inspiring and complicated. During most of my career he had been on the road and gone for weeks at a time. This time afforded me the opportunity to take continuing education classes and study advanced anatomy and kinesiology. In addition to my studies in yoga, I was able to increase my knowledge base with 500 more hours of continuing education in massage and bodywork.

In 2002, I relocated to Las Vegas. I was excited for all the opportunities I would have for growth and new experiences. Las Vegas was the perfect fit for a musician and a massage therapist. The change in location was great for me because I could make a living doing creative work and continue the passion I had for my art. I found many new challenges in my career. The first job that I found was working for a hotel spa doing ten-hour shifts of massage. Next, I found jobs teaching massage to students at a massage school and teaching yoga at a wellness center. After this opportunity, I worked in a well-known spa on the Las Vegas Strip and learned many new modalities while obtaining more professionalism.

In late 2006, I decided I wanted to explore life on my own in Las Vegas and I went through a lot of changes mentally and emotionally. It was challenging, but I learned to stay present and grounded while working and caring compassionately for others. I realized that emotions can affect everyone, including therapists, and these emotions can have an effect on the physical level as well as the mental.

More recently, I have healed from a repetitive stress injury in my feet and ankles in conjunction with a low back injury that was caused from doing barefoot deep compression therapy. This was my favorite massage to perform but I had to learn first hand that repetitive strain injury does not discriminate and it can also happen in the lower extremities. It was a long, hard road to healing this injury but I feel grateful to have had the time to write this book and pleased that I will help many therapists in this field. I have compiled abundant information and ten years of practical experience that has finally come together. Now, I am excited and ready to present this wealth of knowledge to you.

My personal quest is to teach all therapists how to lengthen their careers and keep their passion alive. The career of a bodyworker is very physical and awareness of each of your physical strengths and weaknesses is essential. In this book, you will learn many self-care strategies and safety tips to avoid developing a repetitive stress injury. This book will integrate personal knowledge with professional techniques and it will guide you in the direction of a healthy and injury-free career.

Chapter One

Reasons to Have Proper Body Mechanics

Hands on therapy for healing is one of the oldest healing methods around. The profession of massage therapy became official in 1943 as therapists banded together in Chicago to form the American Massage Therapy Association (AMTA). The 1960's and 1970's showed further interest in health promotion and massage and in the beginning of the 1980's and thereafter, development in the varieties of massage and bodywork grew to over 80 different forms. The phrase "bodywork" developed as a general term and now is used to integrate various forms of manipulation and massage. A survey in The New England Journal of Medicine in January of 1993 acknowledged that massage therapy ranked third among the most frequently used forms of alternative health care. The AMTA is one of the fastest growing health providers in this country. More recently, the business of massage has become substantial. In fact, the Associated Massage & Bodywork Professionals (ABMP) estimated that in January of 2006, 241,058 professionally trained therapists provided massage and bodywork in the United States.

Are you currently in or wanting to start a career in the massage therapy field so you can have a more rewarding career, or so that you can help people? Are you looking for a career that offers you more time and money? Some of the reasons people are drawn to this career are the very same reasons why they burnout or leave the field. When you balance the physical, emotional, and monetary areas of the business, you can have a successful career. When you find balance in your life, you will find that you will be doing what you love, controlling your own destiny, and helping people at the same time.

The truth about a career in the manual therapies is that it is strenuous and physically demanding on your body. You must have strength, endurance, and coordination to accomplish a bodywork session. In the past, massage was an integrated system using movement, exercise, and manual manipulation. It was seldom delivered for a full hour, which is the standard today. To maintain financial stability, most therapists have to complete five, one-hour sessions a day. A recent study in The Journal of Bodywork and Movement Therapies acknowledges that professional massage therapists have a very high percentage of work-related injuries. It is noted that around 78 percent of therapists have had at least one injury in their career and a therapist in the manual therapy field will work for an average of three years and then drop out due to a work-related injury.

Employers need to realize that a day of performing massage is not like most normal eight-hour jobs. Bodyworkers are athletes and the physical work they do takes endurance and strength. Professional athletes do not perform their sport for eight hours a day. Why would we ask bodyworkers to perform for this many hours? Each person is individual and has his/her own unique physical limitations. A large number of bodyworkers push their bodies past what is reasonable and safe. Employers need to encourage their employees to step up when they are experiencing symptoms instead of ignoring them and working through them, which can lead to injury. Employers should realize that injury rates are high for this profession and know that injuries do occur. The employers need to allow employees to cut down on their workload, receive proper treatment, and give them time to rest and heal. Also, they should make sure that the working environment is spacious and ergonomically correct and pay attention to what each employee's limits are and give them enough time in between appointments to reduce injury. When an employee is feeling symptoms in a certain body part, this person needs to be removed from the modality until the symptoms subside. If an employee is experiencing tingling, numbness, or burning, take him/her off of work completely until the symptoms have resolved to avoid a long-term injury. Employers need to take responsibility for the worker, even if the employee does not want to take time off. Sometimes bodyworkers do not know what is best for them at the time and do not realize how much damage has already been done when the symptoms have shown up.

We, as employers, educators and therapists alike must do something to help this profession. How massage and bodywork is delivered must be analyzed and changed. Therapists should not hold the idea that the hands are their primary tools. Thinking this way can lead you to injury. Using a variety of your body's tools and appropriate body mechanics to apply compressive forces to the body are essential. Massage should never be made up of only deep tissue techniques. Overtreating a specific area can be intense on the client and strenuous to the therapist. When an area needs extra attention, the therapist should stop and work on it for a couple of minutes. Then, finish up with some long and flushing strokes in that specific area and move on. Learn to shift gears, when necessary. You are limited by the ability of your own body as your instrument.

Physical, emotional, and monetary burnout can occur amongst therapists and bodyworkers. A major reason why a bodyworker will drop out of this profession is due to a work-related injury. When you do a repetitive or strenuous activity over a prolonged period of time, fatigue is likely to set in. Injuries to the muscles, tendons, and ligaments can occur if you do not become an active player in your health and the well-being of your physical body. If you are not physically able to keep up with the demands of this career, the quality of your work and longevity of your career will be affected.

Many people attracted to the helping field really like to give. Therapists give too much and before they realize it, they end up drained and quit enjoying what they do. You forget to nurture and give back to yourself. Massage therapists and bodyworkers should include flexibility, coordination, cardiovascular fitness, and strength training to ensure a long and healthy career. Good posture and alignment are also essential to staying healthy while doing bodywork. Before you can care for your client, you must care for yourself first.

The best time to learn about proper body mechanics is while still in school. Poor body mechanics are less likely to become habits when students learn early during the basics. Also, educators can help with re-education before an injury occurs. Educators can teach students body awareness and how to protect their own health while educating about massage-related injuries. Schools should take the initiative to include a certain number of mandatory hours in proper body positioning and self-care and these courses should be set as a foundation for all other courses to be built on. Educators need to emphasize the important nature of recognizing the early warning signs of a repetitive use injury. These ideas alone could help prevent injuries from occurring and make therapists' careers a lot happier, healthier, and more secure.

Many different types of employment opportunities are available for bodyworkers. A therapist who is self-employed is allowed the freedom to book as many appointments as he/she would like and leave as much time as needed between appointments. However, being self-employed may not offer as many benefits as an employer could. In a spa setting, the therapist could work six to ten hour shifts, depending on the management, and have only five to ten minutes in between treatments. Recently, spa owners have been making better decisions for therapists by scheduling a variety of services to help deter burnout. Education and thinking from the therapists' point of view, instead of only from a business owner's view is a must for spa owners. Keeping the therapist workload varied is also important to maintain health and reduce rates of injury.

The first spa that I worked at in Las Vegas was in a beautiful hotel off the strip and was definitely an eye opener for me. I worked ten-hour shifts, four days a week. Breaks on a busy workday were few and far between. By the end of three months my arms hurt badly and I injured my teres minor and infraspinatus. This situation was quite different from when I owned my own business and would do no more than five hours of massage a day. I decided that I needed to quit working in a spa where I felt like an assembly line worker. Next, I taught massage at Dahan Institute of Massage Studies so I could give my physical body a break. After teaching for a year, I began working at a world-renowned spa that I had always wanted to work for. I worked part-time doing six-hour shifts, four days a week. Later, I received a full-time position working two eight-hour shifts and two nine-hour shifts still on a four-day workweek. I received breaks to sit down and rest or do my cardiovascular exercise. I also had three rest days and plenty of time to replenish and repair myself.

I really enjoyed the work I did at this spa. I learned and performed a variety of bodywork techniques to keep me healthy and focused. These techniques include deep barefoot compression massage, stone massage, Reiki, Craniosacral therapy, and various body treatments. The varied routine helped me to keep up with the full-time, thirty-hour workweek. I could not have lasted as long had it not been for the variety of technique, my excellent management team, and the understanding and respect management gave to each therapist.

Steps to prolong your career include but are not limited to the following:

- Develop your body awareness.
- Identify the sensations of discomfort and make adjustments before an injury occurs.
- Learn to understand the contributing factors leading to an injury and have awareness of how your body feels as it moves.
- Learn yoga stretching techniques to help you feel your body in a relaxed and lengthened state.
- Employ energy techniques to help boost your energy so that you do not feel as drained after a session.
- Nurture yourself by taking care of your own needs first.
- Set healthy boundaries.
- Be aware of the ways you spend your energy.
- Use deep breathing exercises to help get more oxygen to the muscles and the brain so you can function better.
- Learn to take time for rest and renewal of your body.

Remember, if you do not take care of yourself, then you will not have any energy left to take care of your clients.

Chapter Two

What Do Good Body Mechanics Consist Of?

Good body mechanics are made up of constant awareness, and moving and positioning your body in a way that promotes health and prevents any undue stress or injury to the back, neck, arms, and hands. Practicing good body mechanics is essential to keeping your mind, body, and spirit in good health. To be effective as a therapist this awareness needs to be present in all daily activities so you can take appropriate action to safeguard your career.

The human body is intended for movement and range of motion but it is not designed to perform the prolonged compressive forces that are necessary to do bodywork. Correct positioning of the body must be maintained to provide sufficient pressure throughout the session. Generally, a full-time, professional therapist should be capable of performing four to five massages a day. If you are not able to keep up with this pace, it may be time to take a look at your body mechanics, exercise, and stretching routine.

Some general principles of body mechanics are important to remember. Develop your touch first and allow your hands and fingers to become sensitive to touch on all different levels. Train your fingers to feel diverse textures. Work on yourself to see how certain techniques feel to you and perform specific techniques on honest friends to receive feedback. Palpate, assess, and then manipulate the client's tissue. Work at an oblique angle with your pressure, which means working at a forty-five degree angle to stretch the tissue instead of just compressing it. Allow the client's tissue to draw you in and let the tissue react before moving on to another area. Manipulate the tissue gradually and allow the release to occur. Have clear goals of what you want to achieve, an awareness of the depth you are working at, and know your kinesiology. Continuing education classes can be invaluable and help you to develop touch, learn Kinesiology better, and assist you in determining your depth of pressure. Furthermore, you should receive bodywork from proficient therapists to learn different techniques and sensations. You will receive excellent work on your own body and it will pay off for all the hard work you do on others.

Your role as a therapist is to release tension in your client's body. The amount of pressure applied can affect how the client's tissue releases. Many aspects can influence the amount of pressure and effort you use to perform your work. The amount of lubrication, strength, weight, correct biomechanics, speed of stroke, and awareness of the tissue response can all affect the amount of effort you use in your work. Both client and therapist must be able to surrender to the process for the session to be effective and productive. While you are working, you need to pay attention to signals of strain within your own body. If your hands become weak or shaky, it is a sign that you are working too hard and that you need to switch up your working tool.

To think of massage as something you only do with your hands is incorrect. A therapist who uses the hands for a palpation tool and the whole body for most of the pressure is working correctly. Massage is very physical and the muscles of the arms should not be used for long periods of time without taking a break. The arm muscles are not generally aerobic and fatigue easily; however, the large muscles of the legs and hips can function efficiently for many hours at a time. The lower body muscles can produce power at a more minor level of intensity than the muscles of the arms. Therefore, you should utilize the lower body as much as possible to produce power for all massage techniques.

Muscle strength is not the only source available, as body weight can also be utilized by leaning into each stroke. The key to working smart, not hard, is to develop a system that uses maximum power with minimum effort by combining efficient muscle power with body weight and leaning. Performing long strokes, while leaning, is similar to how you would push a heavy object. To accomplish this, you would stand back at the correct distance and extend your arms out in front of you, lean the body weight forward, and push from the legs with the back upright. The result is achieved using very little effort.

Leaning into the client's body with good structural alignment allows for a more fluid technique and feels better for the client. The client can feel you sinking and easing into the tissue. You will gain more sensitivity to the tissue beneath you as you gradually move into the tissue. As you lean, gravity does most of the work. The body uses primarily postural muscles to maintain leaning and expends much less energy. Mechanically pushing certainly takes a lot more energy and muscle strength than leaning.

Leverage and leaning are essential to reducing fatigue while doing bodywork. Structural alignment should be used in conjunction to prevent injury. In addition to these principles, you should make sure that your table is set at the appropriate height. Set the table height so the top of the table is at the middle of your index finger when your arm is next to your side. Use this as a general starting point and adjust accordingly for what is right for you. If you are doing deep tissue work, lower the table so it is level with the tips of the middle finger, with your arm at your side. If the table is not at the right height, your body will have to adjust to accommodate the height difference. A table that is too high can create an environment for neck and shoulder pain and can cause you to raise the shoulders. A table that is too elevated creates excessive tension that will translate down into your arms. You can bend your knees and use leverage when a table is low, but if a table is too low and you are bending at your back, you can create low back tension and pain. A therapist with low back problems will need to work with the table at a higher level to keep their posture more erect. A person with shoulder problems may need a lower table to use more of their body weight and less muscular effort. Adjust the table when working on different body parts, as often as necessary. Always make sure you can utilize leaning and leverage to do your work. When the client's body is at the right height, you will feel your body working with ease and much less effort. You can also sit in a chair at the client's head and the feet to conserve your energy. If you are in a seated position, keep your sit bones grounded and your spine straight.

Ergonomics and equipment should be taken into account when refining your technique. Make your workspace fit your body. This principle will allow you room to use good body mechanics. You will typically want three feet of space around all sides of the table. Having enough room equals comfort and more efficiency. Consider the width of the table and whether you will have to lean too much if it is too wide. Try to use invest a table that adjusts to the differences in each technique and body part.

Therapists quickly and continually regulate table height as they work. It is of tremendous importance to use correct tools in your trade and that includes your table. An electric table that you can adjust is a great piece of equipment for your body mechanics. A hydraulic table is a must for full-time therapists. Adjusting table height is valuable for efficiency and keeping the body in a neutral and natural position. The correct table height changes from massage to massage and within a single massage session. Not only do you have to think about the table height, you also have to take into account the client on the table. A female client normally adds up to three inches when lying on the table, whereas, a male client can add up to six inches when he lies on the table. With different positions and techniques that you use, it is possible that a change in table height may be required with some or each technique. If you have a manual adjust table, then consider a small stool or a pair of clogs to slip on or off for different heights that you may need. A hydraulic table is an important investment in a long and healthy career. It will provide you with increased body awareness and your comfort level can also be monitored. Sometimes a slight table adjustment can make a big difference in your comfort level or how much strain is placed on your body during a massage.

Table width should be taken into consideration when picking out a table. A table that is too wide can cause you to bend, reach, and twist more than is needed and can cause increased strain on the low back and shoulders, especially for therapists that are shorter. When you lean over a massage table that is too low or too wide, the muscles of the legs, hips, and low back have to contract to counteract the forces of gravity. As you contract the muscles of the low back, force is focused on the L5-S1 area of the spine. Repeated leaning with force can cause physical injury to the intevertebral discs and put you at risk for damage to the disks.

Good body mechanics are important for injury prevention and make you more mindful of ergonomics so you can adapt your work to fit you. Look for various ways to make changes in equipment, tools, and your work environment to make ergonomics work for you. For example, when you are doing deeper work, lower the massage table so you are able to place your upper body over the client by bending from your hip joints. This will allow you to apply pressure with your whole body weight. All therapists have risk factors for musculoskeletal disorders but the key is to use proper body mechanics, in addition to using correct ergonomics. Adapt your work to fit you and then fit your body to your work.

The weight of a table is important to think about because you may lift a portable table many times a day and sometimes it can be lifted from an awkward position. When carrying a table, the opposing muscles of the low back on the opposite side have to compensate for the load on the one side of the body. This can lead to disc damage due to asymmetrical loading. The key is to lighten the load as much as possible or buy a light table if you do a lot of out-call massage. You can put the face cradle, bolsters, and other equipment in another bag and carry it on the other side of your body to balance out the load. If you do out-call massage, it would be a wise investment to purchase a cart to carry your massage table so you can avoid lifting and carrying your portable massage table. Carrying your massage table without a cart can strain your shoulders and low back. If you do not have a cart then use a carrying case with a shoulder strap that can be crossed over to the other shoulder. This way the weight of the table can be distributed on your shoulder and hip. It is most advisable to save your body and prevent injury by wheeling your table around instead of carrying it to your next appointment.

Proper working distance is important for good body mechanics. If you are at the proper distance while working on your client, your power comes from your weight and the use of gravity. Working too close to a client causes you to use more external muscles instead of stronger, internal energy from the core. Conversely, working too far from a client prevents you from using weight and gravity to assist you in your work. The best working distance is when your back, shoulders, elbows, and wrists are extended and relaxed. Your joints should be extended but not locked. You are at the proper working distance when you can use your legs with horizontal power, body weight for depth, and keep the limbs extended so all power is used efficiently.

Two types of stances are important when doing bodywork. One is the symmetric or horse stance and the other is the asymmetric or archer stance. In symmetric stance, think of riding a horse only the feet will be kept on the ground with the knees slightly bent. Both feet are facing forward and shoulder-width apart. Sink your weight, relax the pelvic bowl, and distribute the weight evenly through your hips, knees, and ankles, as you lift the rib cage and float your shoulders back and down. The horse stance is useful for strokes that do not travel far because the feet are kept relatively stable in this stance. This stance is also helpful for techniques that are executed at the side, facing the body. If more strength is needed for this standing position, bend the knees a little deeper or spread the legs slightly farther apart.

The next stance is the asymmetric or archer stance and is executed with one foot in front of the other, with the back foot laterally rotated at a forty-five degree angle. The front knee is flexed and the back foot is used to execute pressure. The front foot is used for balance and seventy percent of the weight should stay on the back leg and foot. This is a lunge position that looks a lot like warrior pose in yoga and is great for applying pressure with strokes that require leverage. (2.1) You can get more leverage from a longer lever and this is the reason that this stance is excellent for leaning into the body beneath you. The archer stance minimizes stress on the whole body especially if the ear, shoulder, hip, and back heel are in alignment. When you are standing either too close or too far from the table, you can compromise the head to heel alignment and set yourself up for injury. The key to generating power in a stroke is to direct the energy from the feet and legs, up through the body, and out through the hands.

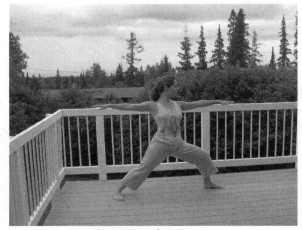

2.1 Warrior Pose

Good body mechanics consist of awareness, effortlessness, motion, examination, restoration and self-care. Awareness has to do with feeling your body kinesthetically during each massage. Kinesthetic awareness gives you a sense of your own movement and offers you a feeling of being alive and three-dimensional. Feeling your body in a kinesthetic way means being there physically in your body and implies that you are aware of how your body is moving in the present moment. Awareness lets the body and mind work together simultaneously. Kinesthetic feeling is process-oriented and makes you experience awareness in the present moment. Awareness influences your physiology and assists your neuromuscular system into functioning more proficiently, in addition to, increasing flexibility and reducing pain. Having a continuous knowledge of your own body performing a massage is fundamental. Awareness on the kinesthetic level shows you that you are living in your body in the present moment. You can experience kinesthetic awareness by feeling your body from the inside to the outside and then allowing all movements to flow. All techniques should go along with attentiveness to prevent a massage from becoming mechanical.

Effortlessness occurs when the performing body moves from a state of ease rather than a state of strain and tension. Your body can do a more efficient job when you work with less effort. If tension is held in your body, it can be transferred to the client's body and can create an atmosphere that is not as easy for them to let go. To work from a state of effortlessness, let your weight distribute over your whole frame. This concept will make using the entire body easier, instead of only using the muscles of the upper extremities. The more you explore and experience from the inside of your body, the better your massage will be. A hurried therapist is more likely to ignore ergonomics and a therapist who is not practicing in the here-and-now is more likely to lock the knees, bend the back, and raise the shoulders. It can be easier to stay with what you know but if that philosophy is no longer working for you, it is time to discover safer and healthier techniques.

Motion is natural and vital to life. The planets move in rhythm with nature. Your heart beats at a certain rate. Your body moves on the macro and micro level. To keep the body moving, a sense of rhythm is needed. Continuous movement is necessary when doing massage and will help you to prevent injury. Any posture that is held for an extended length of time can result in strain, fatigue, and possible injury. When the body is held stable against the table, energy is unnecessarily wasted as upper body strength is solely used. A body in motion, on the other hand, will not get stuck in harmful positions or patterns of strain. As you massage, discover your own style and ride the rhythm like a wave. If you find your body is resting against the table, remind yourself not to lean against the table and keep moving. Keep in mind that movements do not have to be hard or forceful. You should use only the techniques that feel right to your own body. Most people are disconnected from their bodies. Accordingly, it is essential for you to live in your own body and sense what movement feels like from the inside of your physical structure to prevent injury.

Examination contains kinesthetic attentiveness that helps you to self-study your body. What does it feels like to move in your own body? Your body mechanics will improve when you watch yourself giving a massage. Some examples of watching yourself massage are to view yourself in a mirror or your own shadow, videotape yourself, or get a co-worker or instructor to watch you while you work. Give yourself time to be grounded and to be present in the here-and-now. Put some commitment into the space you occupy and set an intention for each massage. Once you are massaging in the present, you will be more aware of the feedback your body gives you.

Proficiency in massage is created from the techniques that you have learned. How you apply these techniques has to do with your skill level, attentiveness, and your creativity. Without continual awareness, you can become mechanical. Always keep an outlook of self-examination without judgment. Self-observation also has to do with feeling pain and realizing that it is as a signal before injury occurs. Think about why your body is giving you a signal and readjust to a more optimal position. Observe yourself without judgment, as you feel where to focus your attention in order to relieve the pain and discomfort. Make time to be aware of the signals your body is giving you and devise a strategy on how to help your body perform with less pain and effort.

Restoration is described as taking time out to revitalize your body. Your body needs time to rest and recover following physical activity and fatigue; it is a must for a healthy career. Pay attention to how your body feels on a daily basis. For example, are you still feeling tired after sleeping, easily distracted, experiencing a change in your mood, or feeling fatigue, pain, or numbness in your body? Save time each day to do something that is relaxing. Take a nap, do yoga or meditation, take a walk, or immerse your body in a warm bath. Give back to yourself at the beginning, middle, and/or end of the day. Consider lying down on your table or the floor and allow your body to rest and unwind, let your palms turn up, keep your heels apart, and relax the whole body as you breathe.

Try gradual muscle relaxation to restore your body. While you are relaxing, tense an area of your body or certain muscles one at a time. After that, release all tension from that area. Contract an area as you inhale and release as you exhale and continue until you have worked the whole body. The technique itself is easy, you just need to tense and release each muscle. This exercise will help you to learn how to identify tension and relax the area before it develops into pain. You can try being more specific by talking to your body and placing your attention on relaxing from head to toe. For instance, tell yourself to relax your scalp, release tension around the jaw, and relax the shoulders as you allow all tension to release from the arms to the hands and out the fingertips. Let the collarbones widen as the chest relaxes and expands, allow the belly to float up and down as tension melts away from the hips to the knees, to the feet and out the tips of the toes. Additionally, you can lay on your back in a comfortable position with your knees bent and feet flat. Let the feet come together as the knees fall out to the sides, place your arms by your sides with the palms up, and allow your back to relax into the ground. Receive your breath like a wave flowing through the entire body, relax and let go, release all your tension, even if it is only momentary. Just a few minutes of rest are effective for total body alignment, relaxation, and renewal. This technique can be practiced any time of the day, especially between clients.

Self-care is a process that has to be ongoing to be effective. When you have finished working on your client, your work is done but your self-care regimen is not over. A regimen of self-care takes place before, during, and after performing a massage. Self-care starts before doing a massage by way of proper nutrition, stretching, and warming up the tissues. During massage, self-care should involve self-awareness, correct body mechanics, and proper table height. After doing massage, self-care continues with stretching, Cryotherapy, and plenty of rest for tissue repair. Life is challenging in many facets and it can be difficult to find the time to care for yourself. A routine of self-care takes time and commitment but it is crucial to the success of your career. Participate in your own health and well-being. Live your life with balance and courage as you integrate your mind, body, and spirit.

Developing body awareness is one of the most important factors to having quality body mechanics. Identifying your own movement habits and feeling the contrast between ease and effort is a choice. You can choose body mechanics that are painful and uncomfortable or you can decide to use your body in a more comfortable and effortless way. The decision to use mechanics that are easier on your body is a constant process. Continual body awareness will help you to develop an inner awareness and a knowledge that will lead you in the direction of a healthy career.

Having good body mechanics includes:

- Body awareness
- Proper positioning of your body
- Applying pressure in the correct way
- Lunging, leaning, and leverage
- Effortlessness
- Examination
- Continuous movement
- Make workspace fit your body

Chapter Three

Preventing Injury by Using Proper Body Mechanics

It is important for you to be aware of the relationship between your body and gravity. Gravity has a big influence in every movement that you make. In order for you to shift your weight and create smooth transitions, you have to be mindful of the effects of gravity on your body. Gravity, base of support, balance, and alignment are all key components to master when performing bodywork.

In the standing position, with both feet together and arms at the side, the center of gravity for most adults is located in the middle of the pelvis, slightly above the navel. The center of gravity can be slightly lower in a female than a male. The center of gravity is the point at which you are in balance and your entire weight is concentrated. Your center of gravity shifts with each movement you make and when the distribution of weight changes, the center of gravity shifts toward greater weight concentration. Some examples of a shift in the center of gravity are moving the arms out in front of your body and your center of gravity will shift slightly forward or if you move one leg out to the to the right side, the center of gravity will have to shift to the right to compensate. Tree Pose in yoga is a great example of using your center of gravity to balance. (3.1)

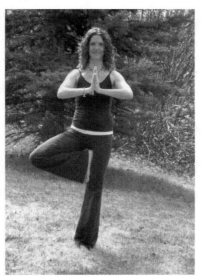
3.1 Tree Pose

Base of support and balance are essential elements to understand when taking into consideration that gravity plays a part on all the movements you make. The base of support is the point of contact with a supporting surface that allows you to oppose the constant force of gravity. Your base of support is the feet when standing and the ischial tuberosities when seated. The base of support is where the point of contact is. Practicing bodywork requires you to keep your base of support over your center of gravity. Balance takes place when your body's center of gravity is maintained over its base of support. "Being in balance" occurs when the body's center of gravity is maintained with respect to the base of support while the body is still or in motion. Balance adjustments, when doing bodywork, can be small but they can make a big difference in the comfort level of your body.

Balance and movement come from proprioception of the body. Proprioception is the unconscious perception of movement of where one's body is in space and involves estimation of weight, force, and effort. This perception allows you to know where your body is in space without having to look or feel. When you are trying to figure out a stroke or sequence of strokes, you are using your sense of proprioception. The muscles, tendons and joints are filled with proprioceptors and can sense pressure, weight, joint position, movement, and musculoskeletal force. When you create a stroke, you feel and subsequently know how much force and speed to apply. Your nervous system constantly monitors your position, calculates essential corrections, and directs adjustments. Signals are sent to the brain, the messages are interpreted, and then the signals are sent as commands back to the muscles. This wonderful system of proprioception helps to keep you in balance and allows you to move gracefully.

The three essential elements of balance are alignment, strength and attention. Alignment is a fundamental piece to possessing correct body mechanics. Alignment is the relationship of the skeleton to the line of gravity and the base of support. The body must be aligned with gravity to be in balance. When you are balanced, you align your body's center of gravity with the earth's gravitational field which puts you in physical equilibrium with the basic forces of nature. Constant awareness of your center of gravity is necessary because you are frequently shifting your weight and recentering your body.

Alignment of your bones is essential when doing massage because less muscle strength is required. The strength that comes from your muscles is used to move the bones into position, hold them in place, and reposition them as needed. When you become skilled at using your bone structure to support your weight, you will waste less muscle energy and effort. Learn to place your center of gravity in the most favorable position so you can conserve energy while using good alignment instead of force.

Use the skeleton to align the body by lining up the bones through the framework and not the muscles. All muscles should be balanced on the bone. Proper alignment occurs when you are balanced and supported, starting with the feet and the legs. Skeletal alignment is essential to having good body mechanics because the skeleton is designed to support your body against the effects of gravity. The body works best when the bone structure is vertically aligned and stacked. Experiencing full awareness of how your body is positioned makes it easier to work with gravity instead of against it.

Think of mountain pose or Tadasana in yoga as an example to explore the fundamentals of a proper foundation. (3.2) In mountain pose, start with your foundation as your origin of stability and balance. Your attention will start at your feet and you should feel the ball, heel, and edges of each foot pressing down into the mat while both arches are lifting up. Lift the toes off the mat, spread them wide, elongate them, and let them press back down into the mat. Be aware that distributing your weight evenly across your feet is crucial to correct alignment. Feel your weight balance on both feet as you let your concentration rise up through the body. Look down to see if your second toe, shin, and knee are in alignment and sense the energy rising as you activate and energize the muscles in your legs without contracting or tensing. You will be pushing down into the ground to lift up. Once the feet are in place, you can apply the four elements of positioning with your hips.

In mountain pose, you will want to equalize hip height, neutralize pelvic tilt, counterbalance front-to-back positioning, and point the pelvis straight ahead. The hip joints should be at the same height when the pelvis is centered over the feet. If you are symmetrical from left to right, your feet will bear equal weight when the pelvis is centered over your foundation. If you are unsure of your placement, shift your pelvis from the left to the right until you feel the same weight on both of your feet. To place your pelvis in neutral alignment, place your fingers on both of your ASIS (anterior superior iliac spines) and sense where your pubic symphysis is. The pubic symphysis and the ASIS should line up on the same vertical plane. The front-to-back position can be felt by shifting the body to the front to feel the sensation of stretch that goes along with the adjustment and by shifting the hips to the back to feel the stretch in the front of the hip disappear. You can also place the palm of one hand on the lower abdomen and the back of the other hand on the sacrum. Rock the pelvis back and forth until you establish a neutral position wherein the base of the pelvis is parallel with the floor. Be aware of the center point and feel the neutral sensation from front-to-back for optimal positioning of the pelvis. The pelvis should be pointing straight ahead when you are in mountain pose without turning the pelvis to one side or the other. Feel for neutral position of the pelvis as you feel the chest rise, the heart open, and the spine lengthen upward. Next, roll the shoulders back and down as you feel the chin become level with the floor. You should have a sense of the back of the neck lengthening and you should always have room to fit an apple in between your chin and your chest. Feel the spine in its natural and neutral position to keep the central channel of the body open for energy to flow. Finally, sense the head floating on top of your body and experience the feeling of a strong foundation with your energy flowing upward.

The outward expression of mountain pose is true alignment of the body from the feet to the top of the head. The internal expression should feel like all body parts are stacked on top of each other. When you are able to feel correct alignment in mountain pose, you will become more empowered and you will learn how to keep your body aligned for a lifetime. Mountain pose is a basic pose that all of the principles of body mechanics can be built off of. Once you learn how to feel from the inside out, you will be able to translate this to your bodywork and have a deeper understanding of alignment.

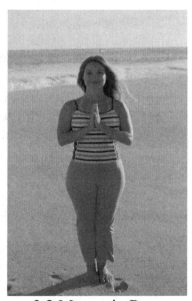
3.2 Mountain Pose

Did you know that the two feet together contain a quarter of all the bones in the human body? The feet are the foundation for the entire weight of the body! Each foot contains 26 bones, 33 muscles, 31 joints, and over 100 ligaments. Your feet are both complex and valuable components of your body. The feet are your body's foundation and the tools for your mobility. Your feet are your connection to the ground and although this foundation is not static like a building, it is strong and flexible with the ability of being mobile. If the base or foundation is not balanced, misalignments will be reflected up through the body. The feet tell your story. They give information about the ankles and the knees and add knowledge about the hips and pelvis. If one of your feet is everted, then the ankle, the knee and sometimes the entire pelvis can be rotated. Give your feet the appreciation they deserve by strengthening, stretching, and wearing properly fitted shoes. Consider getting arch supports from your podiatrist if your arches are flat or overpronated to ensure proper foundation from which your body can work. Therapists stand for many hours a day and next to the hands, the feet are the most important part of your body for support and generation of power. Your body reflects the health of your feet. Happy and healthy feet will result in a happy and healthy body. Think to yourself, when I evenly distribute my weight on both feet, I position myself for proper alignment.

The average head weighs around 15 pounds and its center of gravity is in front of the spine. The muscles in the back of your neck are in contraction most of the time, to hold your head up. You can decrease some of the muscular tension in the posterior part of the neck by balancing your head over your shoulders while standing. This concept is very important for you as a therapist to understand because the amount of stress and fatigue in the neck can be great after a day of holding your head in the wrong position. Forward head posture is very common in this field because you tend to bring your head forward to meet the area you are concentrating on. When the head is held in a forward position the levator scapulae and upper trapezius contract, compromising the flexibility and integrity of the cervical spine. The lower extremities should ground your entire body as the pelvis centers and the spine lifts the body. You should bring the body forward under the head, not the other way around. The head is to be supported by the entire body and your goal should be to reduce the amount of tension while sitting or standing by focusing on balancing your head over your shoulders. Where's your head? Next time you massage, feel where your head is in space. Is it in the middle or forward of your spine? The head's natural center of gravity is only slightly in front of the spine. You need to be fully aware of your head falling too far forward while you work because if your head is held in a forward head posture, the muscles in the back of the neck can become very tense.

Remain vertical and upright when you are standing and feel like the string of a balloon is pulling your head up toward the sky. Imagine the string dropping through the center of the head, down the spine, and through the joints of the hips, knees, and feet. Think of the string as a plumb line to align the head with the spine and down to the feet. (3.3)

Many actions must be coordinated when you are performing bodywork. You must keep your center of gravity over your base of support, which requires diligence and continued awareness. The sensory input you receive from your body can tell you if your body is positioned correctly or incorrectly at the time. As you perform your work, slowly and mindfully, you must focus your attention on your bone and muscle structure and the alignment of your hips and feet. This awareness lends valuable information for when to adjust your body to a more comfortable position. Understanding the balance of how to achieve maximum efficiency while you work and adjusting your body to a more optimal position can be challenging. Performing bodywork requires you "to be in the moment", with a constant focus of attention on your body alignment and how you are applying pressure to each client's body. Attention moves in two basic directions: outward to the world of energy and movement and inward to your thoughts. Keep both directions of attention in balance and you will achieve focused attention on your body as well as, your client's body. Consequently, awareness, alignment and correct body positioning are essential and basic for performing bodywork and keeping your body at peak performance.

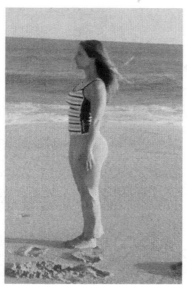

3.3 Side Mountain Pose
Balance the head over the shoulders

Injuries can be prevented with correct alignment of the body, starting with pelvis and hip alignment. Archer stance is a great way to deliver pressure if you are correctly aligned. (3.4) Misalignment can occur in archer stance when the hip of the back leg is pulled too far back or when the hips are not centered over the body. (3.5)

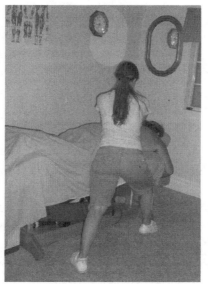

3.4 Correct Archer Stance

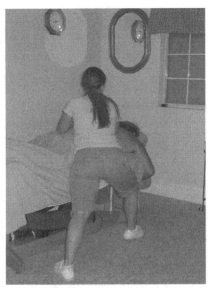
3.5 Incorrect Archer stance

This position reduces skeletal support and makes the muscles work harder. Misalignment disrupts your power and energy because energy does not flow easily through the skeleton with a broken line. Naturally, the hips are to be set under the spine and the body is to be vertically aligned. To be in correct alignment, lengthen and elongate your spine as you slightly tuck in your hips and activate your abdomen. The hips and spine need to be on the same plane to rotate efficiently along the vertical axis. If the hips remain loose and fluid, the energy and power will be translated up through the body easier. With this technique, less downward pressure will be placed on the hip joints, the low back, and the knees.

Counterbalance your pelvis and head to keep the center of gravity over your legs and feet. With this type of balance, you can move liberally and let the upper torso facilitate your work with less effort. When your feet are hip width apart, counterbalancing permits your knees to align over your feet as you balance on one foot and move off the other foot; this gives your stroke three-dimensionality. Surfers know how to ride a wave by bending and counterbalancing their weight. As a surfer rides a wave, he bends from his hip joints and counterbalances the weight of his head and pelvis over his legs and feet. This action allows the upper body to be flexible and gives him the ability move his upper body freely.

Bending over as you massage can become painful if done incorrectly. Your hip joints are the strongest and most stable joints that connect your upper and lower body. When you bend from your "true" hip joints, you engage the strong and powerful muscles from the pelvis and hips. (3.6) Your hip joints support your weight and assist the act of bending while relieving muscular effort of the back and decreasing stress on the spine. However, when you bend from your "false" hip joints or your back, you hang the weight of the head and upper body from the bending point of the spine. (3.7) This action creates excessive strain on the erectors and other muscles of the back. While bending from the back instead of the hip joints, the skeleton is not being used in the most advantageous position and your posterior muscles must compensate for the lack of support. When you bend from your "true" hip joints, it is important to remember to move the pelvis backward slightly and counterbalance the weight of the head and torso over the pelvis. Bend from your "true" hip joints, not from your back or "false" hip joints, and allow your low back to stay flexible and neutral. The knees should stay over and in line with the feet when bending to increase the support from the skeleton and decrease the stress in the knee joints. If not structurally supported, the muscles, tendons, ligaments, and joints can be overly stressed by working hard to maintain stability. Permit your skeleton to do the work for stability and proper alignment. If you bend over a lot during your work, always bend from your "true" hip joints and counteract flexion of the trunk with some gentle extension of the spine throughout your day.

A crucial component of bodywork is to move your arms and hands in synchronization with your entire body. To decrease stress on the arms and effectively perform bodywork, you must coordinate the arms and hands to integrate each movement. When your arms and hands move together with the upper and lower body, your upper body is free and able to allow each movement to be applied in a more effortless manner. The shoulder girdle should hang freely and swing from your torso. The scapula is very mobile and allows the shoulder joint to have a wide range of motion and the ability to achieve complex actions.

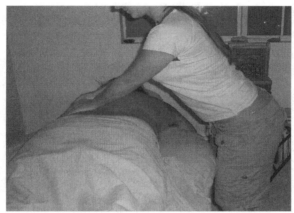
3.6 Bending From True Hip Joints

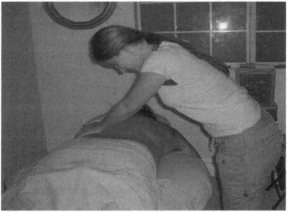
3.7 Bending From False Hip Joints

Since the shoulder joint has such an ability of complex movements and lacks bony attachments, it is important to stabilize each scapula at all times. (3.8) If the scapula is not stabilized, then excess tension can be found in the upper fibers of the trapezius, levator scapulae, rhomboids, infraspinatus, and teres minor, along with various other muscles. (3.9) The scapulas are called on to stabilize and handle the load for the upper extremities activity and movement. Scapular stabilization is a useful technique that keeps your shoulder blades and back in a neutral position. This technique uses the larger muscles of the back for stability. The scapula is the link between the arm and spine, and the muscles of the chest, upper arm, and back attach to the scapula. To stabilize the spine, you must get your scapulas into a neutral position. When this type of stabilization is achieved, you are able to take stress off the arms and feel more of a connection from the arms to the rest of the body. This technique offers you mobility to move the arms with the whole body. To stabilize the scapula you must relax your shoulders and lift the rib cage slightly as you gently slide your scapulas down into a V-shape towards your low back. Sense some width across your shoulder girdle as you envision the scapulas lying flat against the rib cage. The action of depressing the scapula makes the lower trapezius contract and this movement makes the larger muscles provide the support and stability. When working, your scapulas should move along with the arms and maintain a sense of stability as they glide smoothly without winging or lifting off the rib cage. Scapular stabilization should be used with every stroke and should be established prior to each movement. Scapular stabilization will also bring awareness to support proper head and neck placement.

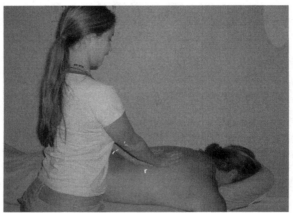

3.8 Stabilized Scapula

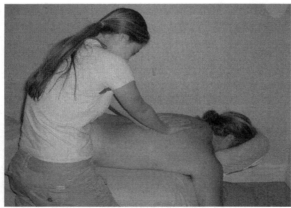

3.9 Unstabilized Scapula

Check your alignment in a mirror. Are your joints stacked? Where's your head? Are your shoulders anteriorly rotated? As you massage, try to develop awareness of where your scapulas are. A neutral shoulder position may feel different to you, but raising the shoulders can cause rotator cuff injury and internal rotation of the shoulders can cause nerve impingement. In time, scapular stabilization will strengthen the lower trapezius and rhomboids, and neutral shoulder position will become easy for you. Now lift your arms and move them around with your scapulas stabilized as you translate this concept into your work.

As you carry out your bodywork, keep moving from one foot to the other as you press your feet down into the ground. This movement allows for fluidity and helps the body to experience less fatigue. A very common mistake is to grip with your feet and use tension to support yourself when executing power strokes. Ground your energy, relax your feet, and keep a connection with the earth. This thought can alleviate you from gripping the ground and translating tension up from your feet. Be aware of your body leaning against the table because it brings your pelvis forward and limits the movement to your upper body. This action will also create tension in your hamstrings and buttocks and forces the upper body to use extra effort to create each stroke.

Continue moving your whole body for every stroke. If you feel stuck, experience which part of your body is not moving. Sink into the tissue beneath you and face your body in the direction of each stroke. Use your hipbones or anterior superior iliac spines as headlights in the direction of the body part you are working on. Drop your weight so you have spring in your legs and let the knees gently flex as you use them to raise and lower the body. Push from the lower body to generate power for each stroke and to increase pressure to the body beneath you as you use your body weight to lunge, lean, and use leverage.

Visualize where you want your hands to go and give each stroke intention. Always work from your core, it is the most efficient point to work from and the most powerful place to generate motion. Try a class in martial arts, tai chi, or chi gong to find your center or dan tien. Power is generated from this area right below the navel; take the power generated and execute whole body strokes. If you feel your energy level drop, simply pull your energy back to your center, breathe, and see yourself grounded. Imagine roots from your feet through the ground. Always start your day with some stretching and breathing to ground yourself for the workday. Grounding is a feeling of being present, relaxed, and balanced, and being rooted into the ground allows your heart to be more open. When you are grounded, your body will feel stronger and more stable. Think to yourself, I am grounded when I feel light, energetic, focused, and work with an open heart.

Perform your work with ease, grace, and effortlessness for the most efficiency. Practicing bodywork with ease becomes apparent when you apply pressure through skeletal alignment with the least amount of strength. You must learn to transfer the power through your hands from the lower body as you keep your weight underneath you and apply pressure slowly and sensitively. Practicing bodywork with grace incorporates fluidity in movement. Dance with the body on the table and move your whole body, not just your hands. Instead of locking your knees, keep them fluid and springy as you make gravity work for you. When you practice bodywork with a sense of effortlessness it means using the least amount of force possible. In contrast, effort is the use of mental or physical energy, often in considerable quantities, in order to achieve a particular goal. Energy and effort will be used as you do bodywork but you will learn to conserve your energy by working with less effort. Learn how to work in a relaxed manner as you pay attention to where your shoulders are and leave them out of the stroke. If an area of your body is under tension, the transfer of energy will be blocked and you will compromise your joints. If the joints are aligned and stacked, energy moves through the body in a straight line and allows you to work with much less effort.

If you feel pain, change your technique to one that feels more comfortable and avoid any technique that creates excess tension and pain. Pain teaches us what techniques to avoid. When something is not in alignment, you will eventually feel pain. Use pain as a signal and readjust your positioning. Ignoring your pain can lead to injury. I ignored the pain in my lower back, which eventually led to an injury. Unknowingly, I was applying pressure while twisting my low back. Twisting while you are applying pressure is one of the most common ways to injure the low back. If I would have listened to my body and readjusted to a position that was more efficient I would not have caused as much damage. The only problem was that I did not know how to adjust my body properly and I continued to ignore the pain. My body locked up on me in order to get my attention and I was forced to start feeling my body. If I would not have changed the position that was causing my pain, I may have had to quit my career as a bodyworker.

First, acknowledge the pain when you feel a sensation that is not comfortable (Awareness). Second, try to trace where the pain is coming from (Source). Third, readjust and try to fix the problem (Solve). You can then start to fix the problem before it becomes an injury or chronic problem. It is essential to constantly have awareness of how your body is operating and know where you are blocking energy.

Furthermore, be aware of the principles of gravity, alignment, balance, base of support, and awareness while you perform your work. Always work with ease, grace, and effortlessness for most efficiency and if you feel pain acknowledge it and adjust to a more optimal position for comfort. Generate power from your core and visualize what you want to accomplish in each session you carry out.

Always create an intention for the session, in addition to the specific work you are performing. Remember, energy follows thought. If you set the intention to release a specific muscle, the outcome is more effortless than if you do not set an intention for the outcome. Focused attention creates a clear flow of energy with each stroke. Negative thoughts can pull you into your head. The intention you set for your work allows energy to be transferred in an unbroken line with specific intention. Think of joy, love, and happiness. Make yourself a vessel of loving and healing energy. A client will feel the difference. Stay in your heart and do not give all your energy away. Keep centered, nurture yourself, and then assist your client.

Get out of your head, get out of your hands, and get into the awareness of your whole body.

Periodically check in with yourself and access your mechanics:

- Prevent your shoulders from lifting up.
- Keep your wrist in alignment with the rest of the arm.
- Avoid hyperextension of the elbows and wrists.
- Make sure the table height is right for you.
- Keep the pelvis moving and mobile.
- Allow movement in the hamstrings and buttocks.
- Keep the knees springy and slightly bent.
- Deliver whole body strokes.
- Prevent tension in the feet when delivering a stroke.
- Avoid twisting your body while applying pressure.
- Maintain focus and awareness at all times.
- Avoid movements that do not occur from weight shift.
- Ensure that the back foot is lined up with rest of body.

Notes

Chapter 4

Creating Strategies for Different Scenarios

Many different strategies must be devised when it comes to a session in the manual therapy profession. Assessing the client is important to the outcome of each session. During the evaluation of the client, you need to figure out which type of massage will be performed, what techniques will be used, and the combination of strokes that you will utilize to create the session. You must be able to adapt at any time during your massage to either your body or the body on the table. You must think about your body and its movements while performing therapy. Awareness is important with adaptability because you have to think about your body mechanics while you are applying pressure, standing, sitting, bending, lifting, pushing, and pulling. When you massage, you also have to be aware of the strokes you are using and how everything combined feels to you and your client.

Applying pressure is a constant function in any kind of manual therapy. Pain and injury can happen to your body from the incorrect use of pressure and body mechanics. When applying pressure, you must find the most efficient angle of alignment. As you know, skeletal alignment uses the strength of the bones, stacked and aligned, to help the body function correctly. You must learn to use the most efficient angle of alignment by stacking the joints, thus allowing your body weight to be transferred through skeletal support rather than from muscular support. To stack the joints, the shoulder, elbow and wrist should line up and you should feel the support of your joints while you work. If you notice that your joints are unstable, adjust your alignment and feel the skeletal strength increase as muscular exertion decreases. If the joints are stacked, they have integrity and integrity allows energy to move in a straight line. An efficient angle of alignment is one in which you can keep your joints supported and stable and one in which you will feel the strength of your alignment when you apply pressure. The big key when working with alignment is to use the most efficient angle of alignment, especially between the hand, arm, and shoulder, to reduce muscular effort.

In this field, irony exists in the fact that some therapists think that using more muscle strength to work an area is better. Therapists sometimes think that the more tension a client has in their body, the more muscle strength they must use to free the tension. It is difficult to remove tension by applying more tension. To work correctly when you apply pressure, face the area of focus as you slowly use your body weight to lunge and lean. To apply pressure correctly, drop your body weight and sink into the area you are working. Connect your feet with the ground and adjust your pressure by bending slightly in the hip and knee joints. Bending the hips and knees as you sink your weight can help you to generate depth of pressure. Holding or applying static pressure on an area for a minute or a few minutes at a time is common but you must realize that it can create strain and fatigue on your body. You should make it a habit to reduce muscle effort, which decreases strain and fatigue on your body. Keep isometric or static contractions to a minimum and when applying static pressure, make sure you breathe into your whole body as you use your body weight for leverage.

Lifting, pulling, and pushing when performing bodywork should be created by making use of correct body mechanics and proper vertical alignment. The actions utilized in bodywork can cause stress and tension in your body when not accomplished correctly. All of these actions are part of your daily routine when performing manual therapy. You must think about and consider how you will achieve these movements before you do them, especially when lifting a body part.

It is important and necessary for you to learn how to lift in a safe manner to avoid injury. Lifting requires you to keep your back in a neutral position and work close to the weight you are lifting, to decrease effort on your body. If your body is not close enough to the weight for you to retain stability, you may be bending at your back and straining the muscles of the arms and shoulders. When a weight is held away from your body, it can be perceived to be ten times heavier than it really is.

It is a good idea to lift with your legs to utilize the power from the lower body. When using the stronger muscles of the lower body to do the work, you save the upper body and the back from injury. Before you lift, bend from your true hip joints as you use the power of the lower body to lift, and as you lift, press your feet into the ground as you straighten your legs. Raise the body to raise the weight and when you lower the weight, bend your knees and lower to the beginning position. When lifting, start by facing the weight you are lifting and keep your body in vertical alignment as you let the upper body assist the holding of the body part. Stay facing the weight when lifting, reposition yourself, and face your whole body in the direction of movement.

Therapists sometimes start by lifting in the direction of anticipated movement and do not take the time to start off by facing the weight and then rotating themselves to allow the whole body to assist the movement of lifting. Lifting while standing in a rotated or twisted position can cause damage to the vertebrae, disks, and soft tissue of your back from the tremendous strain placed on them. Hold the weight only as long as comfortable for you and rest when needed. If you cannot hold the weight comfortably, ask the client to move closer to you or have them assist with the lifting of their body part. Take as many steps as you need to carry out the movement and face your entire body in the direction of movement. There are alternatives to lifting a body part that is too heavy for you. A few examples would be to place a towel under a client's neck to do supine neck work instead of holding the head or place a small towel under the shoulder when working in the prone position. You can work the shoulder in a supine or side-lying position or ask the client to lift their body part to assist you.

Pushing is a demanding component of any manual therapy, one in which you must transfer your body weight while feeling support of the joints. When you need to apply pressure with strength, the lower body should produce the strength needed. Your hip joints become very important when pushing since you bend from your hip joints while pressing your feet into the ground and press your upper body forward. One of the most important concepts to address is using power from the lower body instead of the upper body to generate power and strength. This reduces your risk of injury especially to the smaller muscles and joints of the upper body. When you are pushing, your feet must always maintain the support of your body weight and your legs must work from the most efficient angle of alignment, reducing muscular effort in the upper body.

Stability and support are important when pushing because if either is compromised, the effectiveness of the pushing will be decreased. To stand in a stable manner, the feet must evenly distribute your weight as you bend from your hip joints and keep the back in vertical alignment. When your feet are pressing down equally and you are generating the strength you need from the lower body, the upper body should be able to relax and assist the movement.

Maintain skeletal alignment when pushing for effectiveness and ease since stress and strain can occur at the site of misalignments. The key to pushing with the least amount of muscular effort is using the lower body to generate power, finding the most efficient angle of alignment, and using skeletal alignment. Let the lower body drive the pushing movement while the upper body pursues and assists the movement.

Pulling is similar to the action of pushing, only in the reverse direction. Most of the time, the action of pushing is easier than pulling. If you keep the same principles in mind that you used for pushing, you will create this action with the same effectiveness. When pulling, remain balanced and support yourself with your feet bearing weight equally as you align your skeleton. Use your whole body to pull. As the lower body supports your weight, press your feet down and pull back with your hands. Again, your feet should do most of the work as the upper body only assists the pulling action. Use your entire body to pull in a powerful and dynamic way, while the back is kept in a neutral position and you coordinate the pressing down of the feet with the pulling of your hands. This concept allows you to feel for slight changes. If you want to change your power when pulling, adjust the pressure of your feet into the ground. When you want more pulling power just press your feet more firmly down into the ground and if you want less power, lighten the pressure of your feet into the ground.

How much you press your feet into the ground dictates how much power you will transmit for the action of pulling. Think of the rowing machine at the gym and visualize how you press into the machine with your feet as you pull back with the upper body simultaneously. Pressing with the feet and pulling with the body will produce the power needed to pull correctly. Keep in mind that pushing and pulling can be used simultaneously or separately when manipulating tissue.

The seated position is a good resting position to do your work from but you still have to be cognizant of your posture. You have to remain vertical over your base of support while seated just as you would when you are standing. When you are seated, your "sit bones" or ischial tuberosities are where the weight of the upper body rests, while the upper thighs support the upper body and your feet give additional support to the upper body and sustain the weight of the legs. The feet, thighs and pelvis mutually provide you a base of support when seated. When you balance your upper body in vertical alignment over the pelvis, hinge from your hip joints to avoid strain on the lower back. Sit with your weight over your pelvis and thighs as you bring your ankles under your knees for skeletal support. Keep your knees at the same height as your hips, and your legs and feet hip width apart to maintain stability and reduce muscular effort. (4.1) The base of support is much lower when you are seated than when standing. As a result, it is important to retain vertical alignment when seated and feel the connection through the pelvis, thighs, and feet. To feel for stability, rock your pelvis back and forth to find where neutral is and sense the point of balance. If you find that you are slouching, try tucking a rolled towel under the lower sacrum to alleviate pressure and keep the ischial tuberosities in contact with the chair. When the upper body moves out of neutral alignment, then your center of gravity shifts away from the base of support. (4.2) On the other hand, while you sit with your back in vertical alignment, the back retains its natural curves and decreases muscle effort.

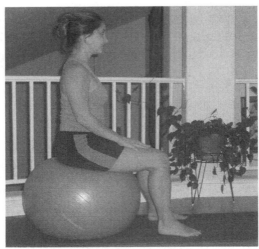

4.1 Correct Seated Posture

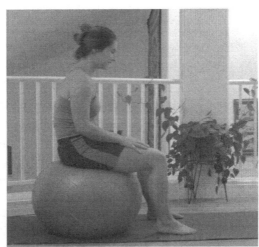

4.2 Incorrect Seated Posture

Sitting in an incorrect way, or slouching, is a major contributor to thoracic outlet and carpal tunnel syndromes and can cause damage to the posterior ligaments and disks of the back. For that reason, while you work in the seated position you should keep your head balanced over your shoulders to avoid any undue strain to the neck. The height of the chair should be low enough to have both of your feet flat on the floor and high enough for you to make use of your upper body weight to generate pressure. A hydraulic chair on wheels is a great investment because you can readjust to the proper height and it is good for ease of use. Working from a seated position can have many advantages for you if done with correct body mechanics and can offer you a break from standing for a few minutes. To apply deeper pressure, you may need to stand since the strength that is needed comes from your lower body.

Now it is time to think about working with the client's positioning. Positioning your client correctly can be advantageous and helps you to reduce stress on your body. Different techniques place you in various positions to your client's body and depend on whether the positioning is prone, supine, or sidelying. Each position can give you access to different parts of the client's body while allowing you the opportunity to work with less effort. I will focus on working with the client in the sidelying position because I feel it is often disregarded as a useful position and it is great for your positioning

40

because you can remain upright with good body alignment. This position gives you the opportunity to bring together the various sections of the body. It only takes a few extra minutes to place a client in the sidelying position. This approach is great for reaching areas that are harder to access from other positions. It is important to be creative in your sessions and working with the sidelying position can be creative and quite effective. You may worry about disrupting your client to reposition them, but you need to do what will be most beneficial for everyone involved. Adapt a style of your own when doing massage from this position. You can use your forearms on the trapezius, erector spinae, latissimus dorsi, quadratus lumborum, gluteal muscles, and the iliotibial band in the sidelying position. This position is also good for low back pain because you can place the pelvis in neutral to reduce pain and access the areas that specifically need to be worked on.

The prone and supine positions are the most common positions to place your client in to do a massage. In the supine position, try to work only on the anterior parts of the body for correct body alignment and less stress on the hands. The supine position can be great for working the anterior thighs and arms, core muscles, and the neck. The prone position is great for working the back, posterior legs and the feet with your hands and forearms. The iliotibial band is the exception when referring to only working the side of the body that is visible to you. The iliotibial band can be worked from either a supine or prone position with a soft fist as your elbow rests against your hip. (4.3) Strategize when thinking about each client's needs and position them appropriately for different techniques.

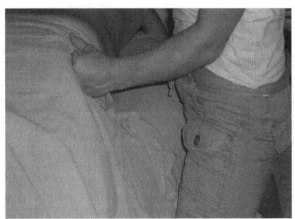
4.3 Elbow against the Hip

Other alternate positions are available to place your client in a more favorable position and to aid in correct body mechanics that puts less stress on your body. Pillows, bolsters, and special cushions can be used to place and prop clients, give added support, and give you accessibility to certain body parts. Properly drape your client for comfort and explain what you are going to achieve. Ask the client to move over to edge of table if you need them to, especially if it will be better for your alignment and efficiency of your technique.

Stretching your client can assist with the release of a muscle and give your hands a break. There are many effective stretches you can do for your client. The neck holds a lot of tension and many stretches could be applied to release this muscle tension. (4.4) (4.5) Also, you can stretch the hamstrings, quadriceps, and calves to give relief to your client. Other various modalities are good to add to your routine. Examples of different techniques to add to your massage are range of motion, joint mobilization, proprioceptive neuromuscular facilitation, and muscle energy technique. Vary your routine and technique and consider complementing your massage with some energy work to facilitate a release. Some examples of various energy modalities to include are Reiki, Craniosacral, and Polarity therapy.

Make sure you have a strategy for each session. Clinical assessment is essential to an intelligent approach in each therapy session. You have to think of many things at once to determine how you will gather information and forge ahead. You must assess the client by looking for patterns of tension, imbalances, restriction in joints and dysfunctional patterns in gait and coordination. Look for balance and patterning to know where you will spend your time and what positioning you will use. Spend 10-15 minutes in one or two different problem areas while still performing a full body massage. Give the client what they want with some detailed work and also give the entire body nurturing for wholeness. Treat the person, not just the site of pain or injury.

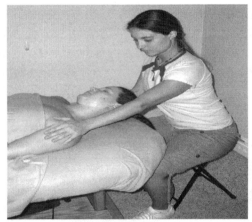
4.4 Neck Stretch

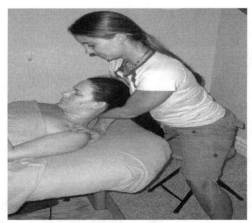
4.5 Neck Stretch

One of the most useful skills you can possess is to know when to concentrate on an area and when it is time to move on. Be careful when you are trying to accomplish too much at a time and know when you have accomplished your goal. Stop and then move on to another area. Working too long in an area that is not ready to release can be painful, waste time, and make the client sore for a few days. If a couple of minutes in an area does not improve or release, develop a new plan or move on to another area. Your well thought-out use of strokes will communicate to the client and allow you to express yourself through your touch. In addition, avoid working in positions that cause you undue stress. Do not limit yourself to specific strokes and techniques or close your mind to new ideas.

Your relationship with your client is very important to the outcome of the session. Treat your client like a person, not a set of symptoms and listen to what they have to say. Provide an environment for healing to occur and maintain a relationship of compassion and trust. The nurturing and healing intention must be present and is very important in massage. Manual therapists, collectively, are generous, compassionate, and nurturing, and are lucky to be able to express these qualities in such a gratifying occupation.

The belief you have about soft tissue is important in how you use your body to apply pressure. Soft tissues of the body respond to touch and when applied in an artful manner, a healing response can occur. Massage therapy and bodywork require a comprehensive knowledge of anatomy and physiology and a variety of approaches to the treatment of soft tissue. Expert knowledge in the bodywork field involves both intuition and intelligence to be successful. You must investigate all possible techniques for manipulation, evaluate the results of your touch, and reevaluate each time you treat a specific body part. The key to manipulating tissue in an artful manner includes using sensitive palpation, understanding how to move through the tissue, and adjusting pressure accordingly.

You must first warm the tissue up and then feel for the point of resistance in that tissue. Determine the readiness of the tissue and respond appropriately. Be sensitive to the tissue dialogue through your palpation and negotiate what kind of pressure is needed to elicit a release. Stress in the soft tissue is a cumulative process and you can use the art of direct tissue manipulation to release the stress that has built up over time.

One of the most important concepts when manipulating soft tissue is to understand that the ground substance of connective tissue can differ from a watery, flexible state to a thick gel-type of state. In some areas of the body, the connective tissue is dense and elastic and in other areas it can be as hard as a rock. Tissue changes can come from dysfunctional movement patterns, trauma, fatigue or injury. Connective tissue becomes colder and more gel-like and loses the capability to stretch when injured or underused. With exercise, stretching, and manipulation of the tissues, the tissue will stay in a more pliable state.

Connective tissue is outstanding in the fact that it is a material that can be altered from a state of thickness to a state of flexibility throughout the body. Connective tissue has the capacity to change from a more fluid state to a thicker, harder state when placed under certain conditions and is possible through thixotropy. Thixotropy is the property of certain fluids to display an alteration in viscosity of the tissues from being hard to soft, depending on what the collagen has been exposed to. Collagen within the deep fascia is a gelatinous substance that organizes itself like that in a quartz crystal. Crystal structures are piezoelectric and can transmit energy when compressed. After working on the client's tissue, you will observe the piezoelectric occurrence when you see the tissue has spread and become more flexible and supple.

Bodywork has a thixotropic effect on tissue and enables a change to take place in the connective tissue from a solid to a more pliable state. Remember there are different states that tissue can be found in and you can assist a change in the tissue to a more pliable state through the use of various bodywork techniques. To reduce the muscular effort on your body when applying pressure, think of your client's tissue like a pillow to sink through, instead of concrete to be blasted through.

One of the greatest joys in life is the potential to express the unique individual that you are. You have to be creative in your work to maintain your enthusiasm. Make use of different tools and techniques to make your work more effective and give your clients the best massage with the finest skills to fulfill each client's needs. Continue improving your anatomical knowledge to allow growth in your area of expertise. Express your individuality to gain confidence. Take a class or learn a new skill. Set yourself apart from others by possessing special skills, through maintaining your interest and passion, and by being the best artist that you can possibly be.

Tips to remember when creating different strategies for a session:

- Use the most efficient angle of alignment to apply pressure.
- Have proper vertical alignment and foot positioning when lifting, pulling, and pushing.
- Let your ischial tuberosities be your base of support when seated.
- Position your client in the best way possible to work most efficiently and effectively.
- Work with the sidelying position in certain cases.
- Have a strategy for each session.
- Have a belief in soft tissue to change into a pliable state.
- Be creative and express yourself when you do your bodywork.

Chapter Five

Refining Your Technique

Technique is a very important aspect for the effects of a session, but what is most important is how you use and deliver each stroke. When refining your technique, it is important to keep in mind that the whole body should be used for each stroke. The whole body is used for applying pressure, transferring weight, and grounding. The upper body comes into play after the power is generated and transferred up from the feet and legs. While performing each technique, your body should be moving just as if you were dancing. The human body functions by laws of motion, especially the law of inertia. If a part of your body is inactive, it will continue in the same manner unless something creates a change. Efficiency can be lost and muscles can fatigue faster if a part of your body is immobile when you are massaging. How you use your body and combine all the tools in your toolbox will make a difference in your effectiveness and efficiency.

A bodyworker will need to combine the following tools to properly perform a massage:

- Grounding
- Weight transfer
- Vectors of force
- The whole body
- Hands
- Forearms
- Elbows
- Techniques
- Diversity of strokes
- Breath

By using the weight of your body more, you use your muscle energy less. If you find yourself using too much muscle power, you can either utilize relaxed leaning or change your foot position to match the direction of force. The most effective way to use your weight is to use the whole body for every stroke. If every movement is a whole body movement, less weight is on the hands and more weight is distributed throughout the entire body.

When you carry out a stroke or technique, take your time and never force your way into the tissue. If you notice you are forcing a stroke, utilize different vectors or directions of force. When you use your body weight properly, the vector of force will be a straight line from your feet to your hands. If this line is broken or misaligned, some part of your body is compromised and working too hard. You may not feel pain immediately if your body is not in alignment; however, repetition of a stroke executed in an incorrect manner can eventually cause injury. The vector of force from your feet to your hands will form an unbroken line if the body is used properly.

Implementing vectors of force and being centered and present can help you to improve your body mechanics tremendously. Being centered implies that you are in balance on a physical level. In addition to remaining centered, moving from your center of gravity can give you more strength and stamina as you carry out your massage. Pressure applied to the client's body is more powerful when originating from your core. Grounding your body keeps your feet connected to the ground and gives you additional strength, moves energy into your core, and is transferred correctly to the arms. When you are in balance with gravity, you have a distributed amount of tension in your body. Learning how to work in a relaxed manner with centering and grounding will facilitate a sense of effortlessness.

Massage uses a force generated forward and downward. When applied correctly, this type of force keeps the weight on the back leg and uses the back foot similar to pressing on a gas pedal to increase pressure. (5.1) The arm generating the pressure should be opposite of the weight bearing leg, which will prevent twisting of the body. Pushing or leaning requires a body that is stable to exert pressure. When you perform a massage, the body should be relaxed, fluid, and balanced. If the weight of the body is on the front foot, then there is no leverage. (5.2) The front, non-weight bearing foot is used to modulate pressure and provide a certain amount of stability. You should be able to pick your front leg up off the floor and still be balanced. The use of leverage, by leaning, is essential to maintaining good body mechanics.

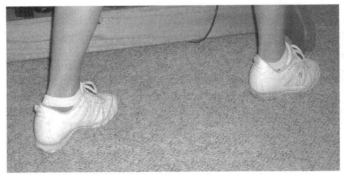
5.1 Correct Foot Placement

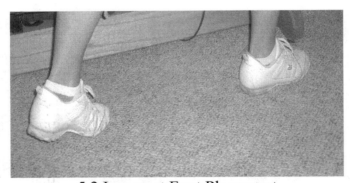
5.2 Incorrect Foot Placement

Depending on the client's position, you can think of using leverage as leaning uphill, or on the contrary, sliding downhill when working on a certain body part. Use leaning, additionally, as an evaluation tool to gather information and feel the resistance in tissue. In a Swedish massage, weight shift occurs while performing the stroke. On the other hand, weight shift will occur before putting your hands on the client and executing the stroke when doing deep tissue massage. Imagine lining yourself up for a pool shot. Focus on where you want your weight to be placed in the early stage of the stroke.

Keep you body behind each stroke. If you find yourself too close to the area you are working on to use your weight and leverage, then take a step back. Compressive force should be applied at no more than a ninety-degree angle in relationship to your body. The client will be positioned so you can lean at an upward angle and you should be able to look down your arm at a forty-five to sixty degree angle. The axillary angle, the angle between your humerus and the side of your body, should not go beyond a ninety-degree angle. (5.3) If your arm is at more than a 90 degree angle, then you are too close to the client's body and need to step back. To uphold the proper angle on a long stroke, walk with the stroke in a smooth manner. Power takes place from using gravity and your own body weight. Think of working at an oblique angle, where the feet and legs supply the force from the ground and the joints are extended but not locked.

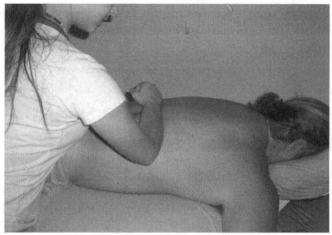
5.3 Axillary Angle

Most massage strokes should be kept at a forty-five to sixty-degree angle in front of you. If the angle is more than sixty degrees, then, most likely, your back is bending and you could be putting yourself at risk for injury. A triangle should form from your hip to your shoulder and to the point of contact on the client. To avoid twisting your body, always keep your navel pointing toward the area you are working on and anytime the direction of movement changes, allow the whole body to change with it. Allow your body to rock and sway with each movement, as you keep the movements slow for fluidity.

Implement this exercise if you find yourself reaching too far on a certain stroke. Tie a rope around your waist to your wrist and make sure the length of the rope allows you to reach out to a forty-five to sixty degree angle. When performing a massage it is necessary to notice where and how your body is positioned. This awareness will prevent you from reaching too far and will pull on your waist when you need to shift or reposition your body. This will give you the tactile experience as you massage to feel the correct length that each stroke should be and how to achieve proper leverage with your body.

I have worked with many massage therapists who perform massage with unnecessary tension. Realize that you can try too hard when it comes to concentrating and controlling your movements and, consequently, you end up restricting your muscles. When you concentrate intensely, you are focusing with effort. When you are first trained to do massage, you concentrate with a reduction of focus on the specific body part or technique. Many actions and processes are happening in your mind and your body when you perform a massage. If you were to only concentrate on your fingers and hands, you would not pay attention to your arms and shoulders, which may be holding extra tension. Awareness helps you to focus without effort and once you expand your awareness, you will hold less stress and tension in your body. Allow your senses to tell you what is going on in and around you by utilizing attentiveness. Awareness then becomes a habitual process of learning how to use your body in an effortless manner and it directs you in the path of least resistance when doing bodywork.

Your session can vary depending on the type, individual person, pressure, speed of stroke, and which body part you use as your tool. You can use many parts of your body for a tool and it all depends on the body part you are working on, what you are trying to achieve, and what is the most comfortable for you. The tool or part of your body you decide to use certainly matters. It is imperative that the tool creates less tension for you while you work and is the most effective and efficient addition to your massage. Using the correct tool will prevent injury to your body and promote efficiency and longevity for your career. The body parts most commonly used for working tools are the fingers, thumb, hand, wrist, knuckles, fist, forearm, and elbow.

When applying pressure, make sure all joints are aligned and support each other. When joints are not aligned, pressure and stress can build up in the areas of misalignment. The more maintained support that comes from the skeleton, the better. Do not apply pressure for long periods of time with any one tool and switch up your tools frequently to keep your body injury-free.

Fingers
The fingers are quite flexible, fairly unstable, and easier to injure than other tools. Fingers provide the hands with dexterity and flexibility. They consist of small bones that are separated by small joints and are joined by ligaments and small muscles. The fingers are made to palpate, grasp and grip, but are not intended to endure a lot of weight bearing. Generally, the fingers are thought of as strong; however, if they are used in weight-bearing ways they can be injured. Therapists use the fingers in various ways: to receive information, palpate, and perform manipulations. The fingers are very important tools to make use of when utilized intelligently. When using the fingers to receive information, use them gently and with lighter pressure. Individually the finger is not very strong, it is better to use a few or all of the fingers together when palpating or applying a technique. The fingers need to be stable at the junction of the hand to work in a correct biomechanical way with the rest of the hand.

When using the fingers keep them relaxed, extended, and slightly bent. The fingers will tend to fatigue more rapidly if kept in a stiff or tight position while manipulating tissue. Apply pressure at an oblique angle as you visualize the tissue stretching beneath your fingers. The fingertips should not be used as a pressure tool because of safety reasons. If you insist on stripping a muscle with your fingertips, you must limit the technique to a few minutes per treatment. The fingers may take some time to build up the strength needed to perform deeper massage. Fingers can be used as a very sensitive tool and while it is okay to use them for deeper work, you should limit their use. Extensor muscles of the forearm are affected by how you make use of your fingers. If the fingers are utilized in a vigorous way, the extensors can become strained. The extensor muscles are also likely to become hypertonic when the fingertips are used repetitively to apply pressure. The flexors can become tight and stressed as a result of manipulating tissue with the fingers in a tense manner. It is quite important to pay close attention to how you use your fingers as you massage. The extensors and flexors can work in balance when the fingers are utilized in a relaxed way.

Fingers are prone to arthritis in the metacarpal joints if used too much for a pressure tool. Always keep the fingers slightly bent and use the soft pads as much as possible. Use a technique called supported fingers by backing up the fingers with the opposite hand (5.4) or with the finger closest to it. (5.5) A good example would be to place the middle finger over the index finger for support when used as a specific tool. The fingers are stronger, stable, and more supported with this technique. With the other hand supporting fingers technique, make sure the fingernails of the massaging hand are completely covered with the supported hand. If at any time the fingers show signs of fatigue or buckle under pressure, it is time to back them up or switch to a stronger tool.

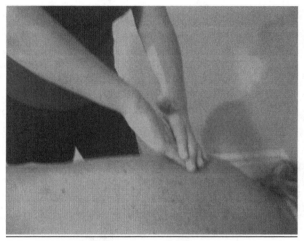
5.4 Supported Fingers

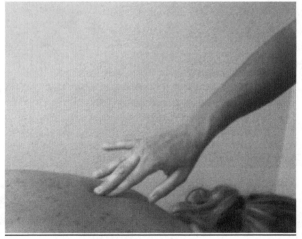
5.5 Supported Finger

Thumb
The thumb has a couple of benefits over the fingers because it has the capability to oppose the fingers, making grasping and gripping possible. The thumb has one less joint and has thick muscles

that connect it to the palm of the hand. The thumb is made up of many muscles, but these muscles are small and fatigue easily. The thumb is a versatile tool but is not to be used as a pressure tool. It is not built for repetitive, compressive forces, especially if pressure is applied over an extensive period of time. For this reason, keep the techniques with your thumbs to a minimum and when using your thumb with your fingers, keep the thumb relaxed.

For every pound of pressure you apply with the thumb, 10-12 pounds of pressure are transferred to the carpal-metacarpal joint. This type of pressure, over a period of time, can create cartilage damage and possible osteoarthritis at the base of the thumb. Pain can be felt at the base of your thumb joint, making it difficult to grasp, grip, and turn objects.

Weight bearing with the thumb can increase your risk of injury. Always back up and support the thumb when in use. If you cannot back the thumb up or support it, it is suggested not to use it. If you feel you have to use the thumb without reinforcement, apply pressure with the joints in alignment and only for a few minutes at a time. Set a limit and stick with the number of times you will use your thumbs in each session.

The healthiest way to use the thumb is to keep it in line with the forearm. One of the most common uses of the thumb is for direct pressure on a trigger point. Feeling and finding a trigger point with the thumb is fine, but once you find the trigger point, place an elbow or a few knuckles on the spot to apply pressure. If you do use the thumb for pressure, back it up and reinforce it with the use of the fingers. A healthy technique is to make a soft fist and let the thumb rest on the index finger as the rest of the fingers wrap around the thumb. (5.6) This technique keeps the thumb in alignment with the arm. Similar to the thumb resting on a soft fist, you can reinforce the thumb by placing it between the index and middle finger when the fingers are made into a soft fist. (5.7)

Another technique, when using the thumb, is to let the whole hand come in contact with the body part while the thumb is in an upright position and the thenar eminence is contacting the body part. With this technique, the hand will move alongside the thumb to provide additional support. (5.8) The arm or leg would be a good place for this technique. Both of these techniques offer reinforcement without using the tip of the thumb and decrease unnecessary pressure on the joint. Some other helpful techniques that include using the thumb are the thumb over thumb technique (5.9) or covered thumb technique. (5.10)

Covered thumb is a very effective way to clear a muscle. Place one completely relaxed hand on the client to use as the tool and place the other hand on top of the thumb with the palm and the fingers resting on the ulnar side of the hand. Compress with the top hand as the bottom hand leads the movement. This technique is a compression clearing method and actually tractions the thumb joint as you work. Areas such as the tibialis anterior, the peroneous muscles, and the vastus lateralis can be cleared with the covered thumb technique. The thumb will face the opposite way that pressure is applied to take extra strain off the thumb. It is important to pay close attention to the wrist and keep it from hyperextending in this position.

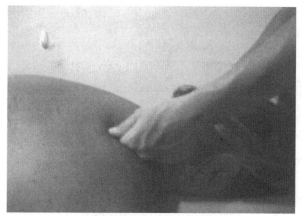
5.6 Thumb with Soft Fist

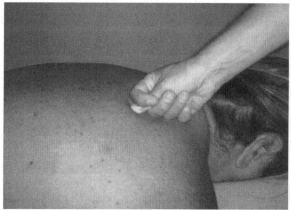
5.7 Supported Thumb between Fingers

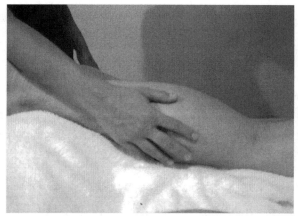
5.8 Whole Hand Supported Thumb

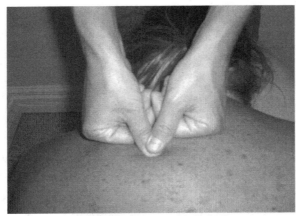

5.9 Thumb over Thumb

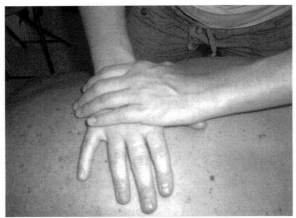

5.10 Covered Thumb

Tendonitis of the muscles that flex the thumb and arthritis are very common and can be incapacitating for the therapist. If the thumb is used for deep work and kept straight, the wrist can be compromised and strain can take place in the soft tissue. What you do today can lay the foundation for injury before symptoms even occur. Once symptoms do arise, it can be too late to undo the damage that has already been done.

Excessive petrissage should be kept to a minimum to reduce strain on the thumb. When applying petrissage, use a closed C approach instead of an open c approach. The closed approach allows you to keep your thumbs close to the fingers and grasp less tissue, which puts less stress on the thumb joint. (5.11) Doing an excessive amount of petrissage can strain the forearm flexors and may result in medial epicondilitis. Save grasping and using the thumb in opposition as a last resort when you feel there are no other options or keep the time you use this motion to a minimum.

Hand
The hand consists of the palm, the heel, and the ulnar blade. The palm is an excellent tool for light and medium types of pressure and can be applied to a broad surface with support of the thumbs and fingers. Each time you use a technique with the palm, keep the wrist and arm in alignment. If you are using both palms at the same time, use both hands equally. The heel of the hand has bony prominences but it is not designed to apply pressure with. The area of the heel where pressure would be applied is where the tendons and nerves pass through the carpal tunnel. Applying pressure only

with the heel of the hand can cause inflammation and injury to the median nerve and tendons. The safest way to use the heel of the hand is to use it in conjunction with the palm and mold your hand to the body. This technique will take the pressure off the area surrounding the carpal tunnel.

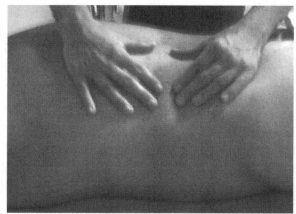
5.11 Closed C Petrissage

Another practical way to use the hand is to use the ulnar side or ulnar blade. (5.12) The ulnar side of the hand is effective for broad pressure areas like the rhomboids, between the shoulder blades. The ulnar blade can be used like a forearm, only on a more minor scale. When applying this technique, keep the wrist in a neutral position. If extra pressure is needed, use the other hand to reinforce and keep the wrist straight.

When using the hands, pair them up if you are able to. This technique is called the hand-over- hand technique. (5.13) You can apply more pressure with the hand-over-hand technique and it can add to the support and stability of the working hand. Keep the hands soft and relaxed as continuous isometric contraction can create a foundation for an overuse of the intrinsic muscles. Hold the thought in your mind that using your hands in a relaxed manner is the healthiest for your body. Tense hands are harmful for your body and are not comfortable for your client either.

Many injuries of the hands are caused from overuse and from using the same motion of the hand over and over. The same muscles and joints can become overworked when used repetitively and can lead to injury and pain. Balanced muscle tone between the flexors and extensors of the wrist is of utmost importance in sustaining health. Be creative and vary the ways you use your hands. Protect your hands and keep them flexible and strong.

Wrist
The wrist is the link between the hand and forearm. In manual therapy, repetitive movements of the wrist are numerous. This structure is more at risk for overuse because it is the connection between the forearm and hand. The wrist is at risk for injury if not held in a stable and aligned position. It is essential to protect your wrists by maintaining hand, wrist, and forearm alignment to diminish recurring stress.

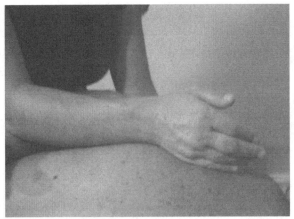

5.12 Ulnar Blade

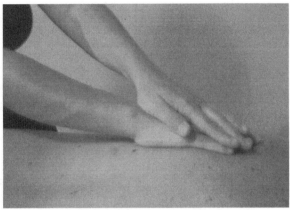

5.13 Hand-over-Hand

Bring attentiveness to the position of your wrists and keep the wrists in a neutral position to avoid hyperextension and radial or ulnar deviation. If you do not keep your attention on the position of your wrists, over time, you can create a bad habit of holding your wrist in deviation. Ulnar and radial deviation can produce a lot of stress on the wrist when held for prolonged periods of time. Ulnar deviation can occur when the arms are held in a pronated position. The body will attempt to create balance from the shoulders internally rotating and the arms abducting with the elbows moving away from the body. This situation can cause ulnar deviation in the wrists and excessive stress on the forearm muscles. You can counteract ulnar deviation by bringing the elbows back to the body and keeping the wrist straight and in a neutral position.

Ulnar deviation often occurs with effleurage strokes, especially when spreading the oil on the back. The most common effleurage stroke, when applying oil around the low back and neck, can cause ulnar deviation. Keep this stroke to a minimum and apply lighter pressure to decrease stress on your wrist. Be careful when holding the wrist in flexion or extension for extended periods of time, especially when applying pressure. Always maintain a neutral position with your wrists to avoid overextending your wrist. Hyperextension is common and sometimes difficult to avoid, but it places a great deal of strain on the structures of the wrist. Discover ways to reduce the angle between your hand and forearm, particularly when applying continual pressure. If you tend to hyperextend your wrists when performing an effleurage stroke around the neck, use less pressure or execute the stroke from the side of the neck to maintain wrist alignment. If you find that your hands or wrists are not straight when you are working then walk your body to the place where your arm and wrist are straight.

When performing stone massage, it is important to pay attention to the wrists. Apply pressure by palming the heated stone instead of gripping it and allow the heat to do the work. (5.14) Envision the stone as an extension of your hand and cup the stone with your palm. Move the stone with slow and moderate pressure and make sure the stone is not too thick or big for your hand. Hyperextension of the wrist is common when doing stone massage. Pay attention to how your wrist is positioned and be aware of any pain in the wrist joint when applying pressure. If the client wants more pressure with this type of massage, try turning the stone on its side and use it as tool to release the muscle. When using a stone as a tool, be conscious of your wrist position. The way to apply deeper pressure with a stone is to place one hand over the top of the other hand to prevent injury to the wrist. (5.15) (5.16) Otherwise, apply only moderate pressure with the stone and let the heat do the work with slow movement. It is not only how you hold the stone, you should also consider the size and shape of the stone and what body part you will be using it on. Generally, match the part of the body with the size of the stone, as long as it fits the size of your hand. You are heating up your own body with this treatment and it is important to stay hydrated and wash your hands in cool water at the completion of the treatment.

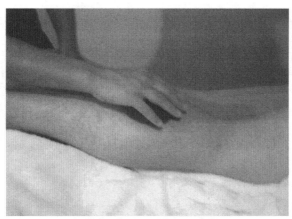
5.14 Palming a Heated Stone

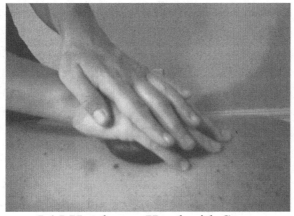
5.15 Hand over Hand with Stone

The best principle to keep in mind when you are using your hands and fingers is to apply pressure with the least amount of effort and strain. Keep the wrists and hands relaxed, as well as long and extended. Envision a zipper extending from the forearm to the palm. If you create deviation with your wrists then the zipper will stick. Keep in mind that tension will always translate from the hands to the wrists, to the elbows, to the shoulders, and then to the neck. The hands, wrists, and fingers all work together to manipulate, grasp and grip tissue, and if used together properly, injury will be less likely to occur.

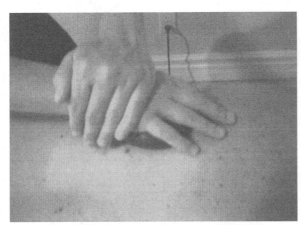
5.16 Hand over Hand with Stone

Knuckles
Most of the time, therapists do not have the strength to use their fingers the entire time when applying deep pressure. You can protect your own body and work with less effort if other body parts are utilized. Direct pressure is better applied with the knuckles, a soft fist, an elbow, or the forearm. The hierarchy of power and strength progresses from the fingers up to the elbow.

The knuckles are great tools to use instead of the fingers and when used in correct alignment they are stronger than the fingers or thumbs. When using the knuckles, use the second and third knuckles or use the second, third, and fourth knuckles together to apply pressure. Try not to use one knuckle alone as a power tool; this can create arthritis in the joint if direct pressure is applied over time. You can cut down on using your thumbs by using the knuckles on the client's hands and feet, instead of the thumbs. Keep the knuckles and wrist straight to transfer power from the arm. Misalignments can create excess strain to both the anterior and posterior aspects of the hand and wrist and the extensor muscle attachments at the lateral epicondyle. A helpful technique when using the knuckles as a power tool is to use supported knuckles by placing the fingers of the other hand around the knuckles with the working wrist in alignment. (5.17) Unlike the fingers, knuckles are used more for general than specific work. If you need to change your angle of use, rotate the shoulder joint instead of the wrist.

The Fist
The fist keeps the fingers safe and permits the hand to become a powerful tool. A fist is formed when the fingers are bent into the palm allowing the use of all four knuckles. The part used for applying pressure is between the phalanges and metacarpals. The fingers are loose and made into a soft fist and the thumb remains relaxed. The elbow should be mostly extended when using the fist. Keep the thumb up and palm facing inward when using the fist to avoid strain on the wrist joint and to keep the wrist in alignment with the elbow and the shoulder. This concept means to make a soft fist with the

thumb relaxed on top, rest the knuckles gently, with the ulnar side of the hand down. (5.18) Be careful not to use continuous deep pressure with the wrist and/or knuckles. A very common mistake can be made when applying pressure with the palm down which can cause the wrist joint to be stressed and hyperextended.

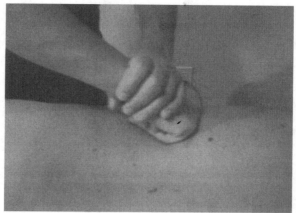

5.17 Supported Knuckles

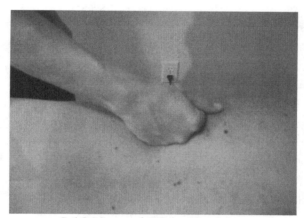

5.18 Neutral Wrist Position

Check your shoulder alignment when using the fist to make sure the shoulder is not raised and to ensure that you are not overusing the muscles of the shoulder girdle. Generally, the table height needs to be slightly lower to use the fist with gravity. The fist is a good tool to work broad and fleshy areas but when deeper pressure and more support are needed, use the fist with the elbow placed against the pelvis. Some good examples of using the fist with support of the elbow placed against the pelvis are working the tensor fascia latae on the lateral part of the leg and around the greater trochanter. The fist is also a valuable tool to use on the arms, hands, legs, and feet at an oblique angle as long as you keep the wrist in a neutral position.

Forearm
The most brilliant way to conserve the energy of your hands is to only use them as needed. The forearm is a helpful tool for broader surface areas. When the wrist is indicating strain or the fist cannot be used correctly, the forearm is a better alternative. Most tissue responds well to the fleshy portion of your forearm and at other times the forearm can be rotated externally to use the ulnar side

as a harder tool. The ulnar area of the forearm is a wise choice to keep the forearm and wrist in a neutral position. (5.19)

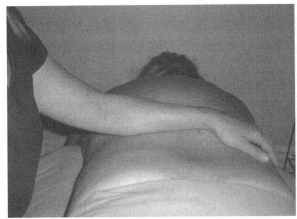

5.19 Neutral Forearm

Use the power that is transferred from the legs to create the stroke and apply pressure closer to the elbow for more proficient transmission of energy. When using the forearm, keep both the hand and wrist relaxed, maintaining a ninety-degree angle at the elbow so the muscles can relax and no energy is lost. Keep the thumb in alignment with the forearm to avoid pronating or supinating the wrist. The action of pronating or supinating the wrist when using the forearm in a weight-bearing position can cause stress on the radioulnar joint. This position can also strain the muscles of the forearm and shoulders. As you work, keep the hand relaxed and be careful not to clench your fist. If you notice that your hand is tense when using your forearm as a tool, breathe, relax, and let go of the tension.

The forearms can substitute for your hands in many techniques. The general movement when using the forearms as a tool is to lunge. Let the movement come from the feet and as you push off the back foot, let the shift of power come from the feet, through the pelvis, and then to the forearm. When small movements or rocking is required, let the same movement begin at your feet. The feet continue to move as you work, as you shift your weight forward and backward. Use a pivot lunge when needed to keep the arms moving on the body or to change positions. The pelvis should be relatively stable as you apply pressure with the forearms and transfer your energy to the upper body. The pelvis will move depending on the size of the stroke and the bigger the movement, the more weight you will transfer from the pelvis. Keep the shoulders and heart space open, while the legs remain relaxed.

Lomi Lomi techniques are very useful on different body parts and are helpful to conserve energy in the hands. As you work with this method, elongate your body and keep the heart open by maintaining openness in the chest as you press off the earth to produce energy. On the back, the forearm can be used in a variety of ways: to warm up the tissue, to prepare and relax the body, to rock the body, and to apply deeper, more steady pressure. You can stretch the tissue by holding one forearm steady and using the other forearm to push the tissue away. Iron the tissue by pressing the fleshy part of the forearm against the tissue while you apply the stroke. You can also alternate both forearms to saw and create friction. When sawing or wringing, use the whole body to create the stroke while you lift your body up to the client's body and drop your body down for a smooth and steady stroke. In the prone position, the forearm can be very useful around the top of the shoulders. To perform this forearm technique, face the client's head and saw from the rhomboids to superior edge of scapula and then use the back of your triceps to pull the tissue back up. When you are working the legs, you can use a compression stroke with the forearm from the hip to the knee. Move slowly into the tissue; sink and melt as the tissue lets you in. The ulnar edge of the forearm can be applied to the lateral edge of the leg. You can also rotate the forearm by pronating and supinating to separate tissue. However, this technique is not one for steady weight bearing. The forearm feels really good on the soles of the feet when the client is prone. You can also use the forearm while the client is supine. You can use the fleshy portion of the forearm on the quadriceps or you can rotate your arm from the ulnar edge to the fleshy part of the forearm to separate individual muscles. In the supine position, you can also work the client's arm with your forearm by gliding from the pectoralis major out to the bicep.

Elbow

While the forearm is used as a broad tool, the elbow is used as a precise tool for smaller areas. An elbow can be used where you would use a thumb, but with more pressure. The elbow is more stable than the thumb, fingers, knuckles, or wrist and helps to reduce overuse of these tools. The part of the elbow that is used is called the olecranon process. This area is good for weight bearing manipulations and for applying specific and sustained pressure. The elbow is very effective with strong and thick tissue that requires specific pressure. To use the elbow, bend the joint to ninety degrees as you relax the forearm and the entire hand. You can either internally rotate the humerus to use the elbow or raise the arm so it is straight up in the air, in a vertical position. Using the elbow with the arm horizontal can be a good alternative to using the hands. (5.20) This can be an effective means to separate muscle tension in areas like the erectors or the hamstrings.

For deeper pressure, raise the arm up, bring the body over the area, and if more pressure is needed, place one hand on top of the other. (5.21) The deeper you work, the slower you should move into the tissue. Always allow the tissue to draw you in. You can also move the client's limb passively with elbow pressure on a specific area to create more depth in the tissue with a pin and stretch technique. The olecranon process can be utilized on the client's palm and sole of the foot for certain trigger points. Only apply pressure with the distal part of the olecranon process and do not use the point of the olecranon process for pressure because the ulnar nerve is not very protected and can be inflamed and possibly damaged. The elbow has less receptivity than other tools but you can sensitize your elbow with time and practice. Palpate with the fingers first and then apply pressure with the elbow. You can also use the other hand to guide the elbow away from any bony structures. To apply pressure correctly with the elbow, use your body weight to lean into the tissue with the scapula stabilized. It is very important, when using the forearm or elbow, to use the lower trapezius to stabilize the scapula and keep the strain off of the shoulder joint. Depressing the shoulder joint rotates the glenohumeral joint downward and brings the shaft of the humerus into alignment with the socket. Relax your elbow while maintaining stability in your shoulder joint. This action will take some of the strain off of the pectoralis minor, lower trapezius, and the latissimus dorsi. Most deep work can be done using the elbow. The elbow is a powerful tool that can achieve big results with minimal effort.

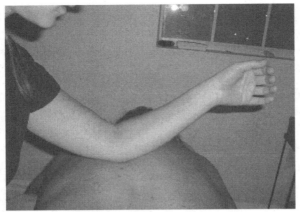
5.20 Horizontal Elbow

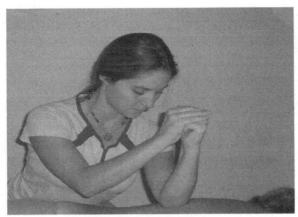
5.21 Vertical Elbow

If you find that a stroke is not working for you, try switching to another tool instead of changing your position. If the method is not working then switch positions entirely. Change your position and switch up your tools as often as necessary. Keep in mind that if you use any tool excessively, you can put yourself at risk for injury. Any muscle used in static contraction over an extended period of time can set you up for injury. The rotator cuff muscles can be overused by having to stabilize the head of the humerus, when using a technique frequently with the forearm or elbow.

Swedish massage is generally executed using lighter pressure and as always, proper body mechanics is important. Lunging and leaning is employed with lighter strokes but with less strength than deeper work. Deep tissue massage uses more strength generated from the lower body and should consist of inertia and melting to release the tissue. The recipe for deep tissue is compression multiplied by time equals the penetration and depth of the tissue. Connect with your client by slowing down while applying pressure. Applying slow and steady pressure is how you can create profound changes in your client's body.

Deeper strokes can sometimes cause discomfort and even pain for your client. Know that there is a line between discomfort and pain. Have the client verbalize what they are feeling and articulate what sensations are felt. A lot of times an intense sensation can be one of pain. Make sure to get feedback from your client and do not exceed a seven on a 1 to 10 scale. Do not knowingly cause pain on your clients. Get the client involved in the process by receiving feedback from them and allowing the client to let go through the process of relaxation. Pain can be the outcome of carrying out a stroke too quickly. A sure sign of excessive pressure or forcing your stroke can be apparent when the client tenses under your hand, forearm, or elbow. If the client can breathe through and receive the pressure with intensity yet stay relaxed, then you know the technique was performed correctly.

Pay attention to your body with each massage stroke that is executed. Many different strokes are combined to carry out a massage. Various strokes of massage are compression, effleurage, petrissage, percussion, friction, and vibration. The compression stroke can be distributed by using the finger pads, fist, forearm, palm or heel of the hand. To apply compression, lean and sink into the tissue beneath you. Only use the fingertips for smaller areas with little tissue. If you are using compression on a larger area or for an extended period of time, place one hand on top of the other.

The basic massage strokes are effleurage, petrissage, tapotement, friction, and vibration. Effleurage means to stroke or touch lightly and is the most utilized massage technique. You can massage the whole body using different speeds and pressures of the basic effleurage stroke. Effleurage can be delivered with the fingertips, palms, knuckles, or forearms. Mold your hand to the body part you are working on and keep the hands and wrists relaxed. Also, keep the joints stacked as you lunge and lean from the feet and legs up. With horizontal stroking, move across the width of the body part and use the legs to execute the movement.

Petrissage is a kneading of the muscle. With this stroke, try to keep the fingers together and scoop the tissue into the fleshy part of the thumb. It is healthier for the thumb to scoop and lift with the fingers instead of grasping and using the thumb do most of the work. Petrissage in this form is challenging because it is requires a lot of muscular effort and should be kept to a minimum. Different forms of petrissage can be performed with a soft fist formed into a cupped hand or an alternate lift and wring.

Tapotement, friction, and vibration are some other basic massage strokes. Percussion or tapotement is a pounding stroke and is stimulating. The main objective with tapotement is to keep the hands and fingers relaxed. Friction is applied mostly with the palms or fingertips. For superficial friction, you need to keep the arms, wrists, and hands relaxed. For deep friction, work perpendicular to the muscle fibers or in a circular motion. Use the fingers, knuckles, or forearms and keep the joints stacked with a proper lean for deep friction. Vibration is better applied with loose and relaxed shoulders, arms, wrists, and hands. Relax your fingertips on the client and move your hand with a soft trembling motion.

Let the hands rest on the tissue and listen as they touch. Always warm up the tissue first to create more suppleness and add rocking to your routine to relax and soften tissue. Make use of the effleurage stroke to connect each stroke and soothe the body. Vibration can be utilized for helping a tense area to relax and release. You can also include stretching and range of motion exercises to lessen the repetitive motion of the hands.

In addition to the hands, massage can also be adapted by using the feet. Deep barefoot compression massage is an excellent technique used for broad, deep-tissue strokes. With this modality, bars are used overhead for support and balance, lubrication is applied, and deep gliding effleurage is used to move smoothly over the body. Gravity assists this compression therapy as the whole body weight is utilized. This type of massage elongates the client's spine and the muscles surrounding it. This massage is mostly performed with the heel and lateral plantar surface of the foot, however, the medial portion of the foot, instep, tarsals, and metatarsals are used as well. This style of massage requires balance, slow, smooth movements, and a relaxed foot and toes to execute the effleurage strokes. The slow, deep pressure stretches the client's muscles and tendons away from the origin and releases the soft tissue, not to mention, it increases movement of blood and lymphatic fluid.

The accomplishment of this type of massage has to do with the application of your body weight and upper arm strength. As a therapist in this modality, you should allow your weight to distribute evenly and leverage the body weight through the feet. Keep the feet soft and relaxed when working and realize that if you work with tense feet, tension will translate up into the muscles of the legs and hips. You will want to feel your muscles and bones through your toes, arch, heel, and every part of your foot when using barefoot compression. Become three-dimensional and perceptive with your feet by feeling with every aspect of your foot. (5.22) Allow gravity to do the work for you as you bend your knees, rotate the hips, and allow your body weight to give the pressure. Coordinate the breath and your body weight to shift effortlessly and generate power from the core of the body, not from the legs alone. Core strength is very important in this modality for balance, power, and strength. Keep the arms at a 90 degree angle above the head when working with the bars. (5.23) Most of your weight is controlled and held in the upper arms depending on the client needs. Stable and steady pressure comes from a line of energy from the hand to the heel and flows from the knee through the foot. If more pressure is needed, you can push against the bars or press against the walls. Just make sure whatever stroke you are using feels right for your body.

Deep barefoot compression massage can reduce your risk of repetitive strain syndrome because you use long, deep strokes with the feet and cover more area which helps to avoid the small, repetitive movements with your hands. You can prevent injury to the low back since less time is spent bending over the body and your body weight is doing the work. Be aware that repetitive strain syndrome can happen in the feet as tarsal tunnel if you use too many small and intricate techniques with the feet. Take every measure possible, notice early warning signs, and seek treatment early if you notice ongoing pain, numbness, burning, or tingling. Ice the feet and ankles if performing more than a few sessions daily and especially if you are feeling pain. Stretch the leg and hip muscles daily, especially the soleus, hamstrings, gastrocnemius, hip rotators and low back muscles. Self-massage and release the trigger points in your low back, gluteals, piriformis, hamstrings, gastrocnemius, soleus, and the tibialis posterior and anterior muscles. Most importantly, the isometric nature of this massage demands that you receive massage often on the lower leg, hip, and back muscles. In addition, since this type of massage demands so much upper arm strength, it is wise to be diligent in stretching the rotator cuff and pectoralis muscles to retain flexibility and also receive massage on your upper body. Regular massage helps to release myofascial adhesions and lengthen the tissue for better range of motion and movement.

In addition to using the tools of your body, you can also supplement by using certain handheld tools for more efficiency. You can help counteract the overuse of your hands by the use of handheld tools. Applying pressure to with the fingertips can lead to inflammation and reduced circulation in the fingertips, in addition to creating pressure in the carpal tunnel area. It is a wise idea to use your hands to find and locate a trigger point or certain adhesions and then switch to a tool. Look for a tool you can grip, in a comfortable way, with all the fingers and the thumb. Avoid a tool that you only grip with your fingertips or one that will put pressure on the palm. A tool should allow you to apply pressure without having pain and should not be relied on but used as a supplement to a massage.

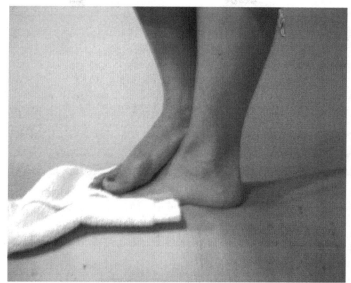
5.22 Three-Dimensional Feet

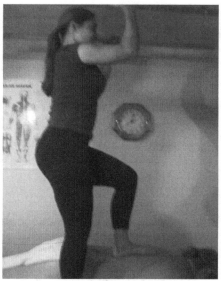
5.23 Arms at 90 Degree Angle

What tool you use depends on what type of massage you are giving, the size of the client, and what the person's needs are. There are many different tools to choose from. You can find anything from a thumb tool to a T-shaped tool to a knob-shaped tool. Educate yourself on each tool before you select one. Make sure your place of employment accepts the use of a tool. Some spas do not allow tools because of the risk of liability. Tools are used generally for clinical work and can be utilized easily from a seated or standing position. When purchasing a handheld tool, take into account the contact surface area of the tool. A broader area of tissue is accessed when using a larger surface area tool. On the other hand, the smaller the area of tissue you are working on, the more precise the instrument needed for proper manipulation. You should choose a tool that suits your modality and techniques. A handheld tool will transfer the force from the joints of your arm and hand to the tool. It is of utmost importance that your joints are stacked and the wrist is not hyperextended when using a tool. Be cautious when using any kind of a tool, get permission, and know your client's contraindications. If you can have a longer and healthier career by supplementing your massage with a tool, in a safe manner, then use the tool of choice with confidence and with caution. Remember that a handheld tool should be used as an extension of your hand to assist you in doing deeper work and will reduce strain on your own body's tissues.

You should develop a wide range of working methods to suit your physical capabilities. It is invaluable to be creative, resourceful, and sensitive to touch. You need to be able to feel subtle responses or changes in the tissue beneath you. Feel for the softening of the tissue and the sinking of your tool of choice. Move on to another area, after the softening and lengthening of the tissue happens. If a stroke is done too quickly, it is more difficult to access if or when the softening happens. Each time a stroke is performed, it is best to work slowly and wait for a melting or softening in the tissue. This explanation has to do with the concept of inertia. To accomplish melting of the tissue, you have to build up the momentum. Start slowly by sinking into the tissue beneath you, allowing the lunging and leaning of body weight to increase as you sink. Once inertia has been accomplished, less force is required because the accumulated effort has taken place. The area manipulated has, in effect, relaxed and let go. Using this method is essential to doing deep massage and preventing overuse injuries.

Many therapists try too hard and think they can work all the tension out at once. Only give the body on the table what it wants at the time. Follow the tissue as far as it will go and when the tissue pushes against you, back out and hold pressure. Respect what is held in the tissue beneath you and you will work with less effort.

Some therapists develop a habit of getting stuck in particular routines and using the same strokes over and over. Certain spa settings can have cookie cutter massages in fifty-minute sessions. Burnout, injury, and loss of enthusiasm can be common if you work in a production line or if you are always performing a set routine. It is essential to think of the client as an individual and have goals for each client and particular massage. Chances of injury are also higher if you are performing the same routine because grounding, centering, and proper body mechanics are usually not being utilized. Being in the moment and using varied techniques is essential to a healthy career.

Points to assist with proper use of your body when performing bodywork:

- Do not get stuck in the same routine.
- Keep the wrist in alignment with the arm.
- Use the tool that is efficient, effective and comfortable for you.
- Let the hands listen and touch as they rest on the body.
- Avoid any techniques that cause pain.
- Switch to a forearm or elbow to do deeper work.
- Apply pressure with the least amount of stress and strain.
- Back up your tool of choice for additional pressure.
- If the technique hurts your body, do not use it.

Remember to work with movements that are smooth and even and shift your body often.

Chapter Six

Anatomy

You can benefit greatly from studying anatomy. The study of anatomy helps you to recognize the landmarks of the body for exceptional palpation skills. As a therapist, you must know and perform skilled palpation for whatever body type you have on the table. Having the knowledge of palpation is important for your confidence and the effectiveness of each session. A therapist that is skilled should have the information and education to know what action each muscle has, how the body works as a whole, and you must be able to devise a plan on where to work on each client's body. Understanding the role of each structure in the body and how everything works together is quite important in this field. As a manual therapist, a quick review of anatomy always works to your advantage because the exploration of the human body is never the same on any two individuals.

The musculoskeletal system is made up of the skeletal system of bones and joints and the skeletal muscle system. This whole system provides form, stability, and movement for the human body. The skeleton is the framework of the body and is made up of many bones. The skeleton provides support for the body and attachment for muscles while storing and manufacturing blood cells in the bone marrow. The musculoskeletal system is accountable for posture, movement, and protection of the organs. It is made up of muscles, bones, tendons, ligaments, and joints. The bones work as levers for the action of muscles. The union of two bones is held together by ligaments and is called a joint. Ligaments function to stabilize and strengthen a joint in a passive manner. Ligaments are strong and tensile and hold bones together and tendons are tough, flexible bands of tissue that attach muscle to bone.

The core of the body consists of the spine, skeleton, and pelvis. It is at the very center of the body and serves as a base while providing stability. The spine channels its weight through the sacrum and into the pelvis. If the pelvis is rotated or tilted, the natural curves can be thrown off and an imbalance can occur. These types of imbalances can affect posture and alignment of the body as well as, muscle balance. Like the spine, the pelvis is an important component in the performance of the entire body and must be balanced in order to initiate movement correctly.

The spine is meant to be flexible and stable at the same time; it allows the body to stabilize itself as it moves. A healthy spine forms three natural curves and extends from the bottom of the buttocks to the base of the skull. The vertebral column can bend and rotate and has twenty-three intevertebral articulations with twenty-four vertebrae. The vertebrae are connected via ligament bands and strong muscle tissue. The spine helps to support the shoulder girdle and the vertebral column protects the spinal cord. Nerve roots exit between small openings in the vertebrae and supply the muscles and organs with sensory information. It is necessary to keep the vertebrae properly aligned and stabilized for proper functioning. The spine needs to be mobile and have space in order for the body to give and receive messages correctly.

The shoulder girdle is made up of the shoulder blades, collarbones, the head of the humerus and three joints. The shoulder is a very mobile joint. The upper body includes the head, neck, upper back, arms, and shoulders. If the head is in alignment on top of the spine, the neck can move freely and less muscle tension is used. When you stand correctly, the arms hang freely, the chest is open, and the hands, fingers, and wrists are relaxed. If the muscles surrounding the shoulders are tense, this tension will translate down into the hands and wrists. The most mobile joint in your body is the shoulder joint, making it less stable and more prone to injury. Stiff shoulders and a rounded back can cause poor posture over time. A habit of rounding the shoulders and tensing the muscles of the shoulders can be corrected with awareness and stretching, and eventually you can restore normal range of motion.

The radius joins with the carpal bones at the wrist and the carpals articulate with the phalanges. The hand is versatile and competent of jobs ranging from precise movements to ones of great strength. The thumb is opposable and allows you to grip and manipulate objects. The carpals consist of eight bones; two of which articulate with the radius. The carpals form an anteriorly concave arch with a thick ligament that covers the tendons and nerves. The carpal tunnel is the space between the carpal arch and the flexor retinaculum. The structure makes up the floor and the walls of the carpal tunnel and the flexor retinaculum forms the roof. This tunnel is a passageway for nine flexor tendons and the median nerve; these nerves and tendons give the hand function, movement, and feeling. The carpal tunnel is a narrow space for the flexor tendons and nerves to pass through and is about the diameter of an index finger. The tendons normally glide past each other; however, when inflammation is present or the size of the tunnel decreases, the median nerve can become impinged.

The hip is a sturdy ball-and-socket joint protected by strong muscles. The ball fits in a socket of the pelvis and the socket of the hips is cushioned with cartilage and ligaments that hold the joint together. The ligaments allow only limited movement for the hip joint. The hip joints are flexible if they can move back and forth and swing across the body. Most people in the western society have tight hips because they sit in chairs. Sitting too much can cause the hips to lose the capability to rotate. Stretching loosens up stiff hips and helps to maintain flexibility.

Fascia is a soft tissue component of connective tissue which is distributed throughout the body in a three dimensional web from head to foot. The fascia is a sheath that surrounds every muscle, bone, nerve, organ, and blood vessel of the body. Fascia unites and wraps all structures with its moist, fibrous cohering sheets and strands, and is considered one of the most complex and extensive organs of the body because of the complexity and continuity. Few organs have such an extraordinary diversity of functions and while connective tissue is basically a moveable structure, it also supports your posture and holds everything in place. Malfunction of the fascial system due to trauma, injury, posture, and inflammation can cause adhesions and result in irregular pressure on the organs, nerves, muscles, and bones. Fascia also creates an environment for healing after an injury has occurred.

Every joint in the body is controlled by different groups of muscles. Certain joints have rotator muscles that rotate the bone and flexor muscles that contract or bend the joint while the extensor muscles straighten the joint. Muscles hold the body upright, maintain posture, and allow the body to create motion. Muscles act as puppet strings that move the skeleton around. Muscles have an active ability to contract and a passive capability because of elasticity. When stretched properly, a healthy muscle can be reset to the normal resting length.

Muscles work together with the skeletal system and the nervous system. Muscles are fundamental to the human body and account for about half of the body's weight. Muscles stretch from one bone to another and attach to bone by tendinous material. Muscles have two ends; one end is a fixed attachment called the origin and the more moveable end of a muscle is called the insertion. Each muscle fiber has its own nerve supply. All voluntary muscles contract when stimulated, relax after contraction, and can be excited by a nerve or stimulus. The middle of the muscle is called the belly and is where each initial contraction takes place. Muscles work by the all-or-nothing response. Either all muscle fibers contract or no contraction happens at all. Oxygen is the fuel of combustion in muscular activity. For that reason, insufficient oxygen supply to the muscle tissue can lead to an accumulation of waste products and can cause muscles to weaken. Muscles generate motion and can also restrict motion; they are arranged into paired opposites. One muscle contracts while the opposite muscle relaxes. As the muscle contracts, it pulls the bones of its attachment in the direction of contraction. When a muscle relaxes, the opposite muscle is allowed to pull the bone the other way. **A muscle cannot push. All muscles pull!**

A shortening action takes place when the muscle contracts and moves the bones closer together. Strength comes from the size of a muscle and its ability to contract, and power comes from the degree of movement the contraction achieves. If a muscle in the relaxing phase does not relax fully, it will have more resistance and create a loss of power and performance. Any muscle that is worked repetitively, in the same range of motion, will shorten. To lengthen a muscle, you should employ some type of stretching. Stretching reduces the risk of injury and keeps the muscles, tendons, ligaments, and connective tissue more flexible. Over time as a muscle tightens, it also becomes weak. Thus, the relaxing phase of the muscle happens slower, but not completely, and will cause the contracting muscle to work harder.

Skeletal muscles serve two different, but important purposes: movement and support. Skeletal muscles move the body through space, produce large spurts of movement with gravity or control tiny, subtle movements, and support the position of the bones in relation to each other. The two types of skeletal muscles are postural and phasic. The postural muscles work to uphold your posture, support the body against the force of gravity and are not easily tired. Postural muscles have many slow-twitch red fibers that can hold a muscle contraction for a while before fatigue sets in. Postural muscles, also known as tonic muscles, are designed for endurance, are workhorse muscles, and sustain a semi-contracted state. Also, postural muscles are slow and steady, need sufficient time to respond, and have a tendency to shorten and become hypertonic when placed under strain. This type of muscle may cramp. Postural muscles take time to respond and do not give quick bursts of strength. Depending on your reference source, the postural muscles can be listed differently. From my research, I found that the postural muscles are the following: the gastocnemius, soleus, medial hamstrings, adductors psoas, piriformis, tensor fascia latae, quadratus lumborum, erector spinae, latissimus dorsi, upper trapezius, sternocleidomastoid, levator scapulae, pectoralis major, and in some cases, the scalenes.

Muscles that support the body against gravity are postural and can produce inefficient neurological patterns, trigger points, build-up in the connective tissue, and can become hypertonic. If your posture is not balanced, postural muscles function like ligaments or bones and extra connective tissue is added to the muscle to give the body more stabilization against gravity. The problem with additional connective tissue build up on a postural muscle is that it becomes more static tissue and is less able to stretch. Since these muscles are voluntary, you have control over the quality of movement when used in a balanced manner. An incorrect usage of postural muscles can lead to excessive tightness and can cause the skeleton to become misaligned. When you develop body awareness, the muscle and skeletal system can work better together. With this balance in power, the postural muscles can move easier without unnecessary tightness and excessive effort.

In contrast to a postural muscle, a phasic muscle requires an attentive decision on your part to contract. The phasic or active muscles are designed more for movement. They are made up of more fast-twitch fibers, are not built for endurance, fatigue quickly, and will not shorten but will become weak. Phasic muscles react quickly, but tire out fast and require more recovery time. Problems in the musculotendinous junction are found more in phasic muscles and become hypertonic mostly from repetitive use or a sudden postural change, such as an accident or trauma. Phasic muscles are gluteus maximus, abdominals, quadriceps, tibialis anterior, biceps, triceps, brachioradialis, and deltoid. Your muscles never work in isolation. If a muscle is too tight it can dominate and disturb the natural movement of a joint. On the other hand, if a muscle is too weak, it can cause the assisting muscles to overwork and also disrupts the natural movement of a joint. Tonic muscles sometimes work even when they are not supposed to and take over for other muscles. Muscle imbalance will not go away unless you stretch and relax the tightened muscles before you strengthen the weaker muscles. If you are sitting at a desk for ten hours, some muscles are being contracted and some muscles are being stretched. When you go to the gym that evening, you would want to stretch the muscles that were contracted all day and then strengthen the weaker, overworked muscles. Muscle imbalance in the body makes the postural muscles weak in response to shortening and as the postural muscles are stretched and lengthened, the phasic muscles become stronger.

Muscles and bones obviously work together and it is important for you as a therapist to know how the musculoskeletal system works collectively to be able to treat the client. The main abnormalities in musculoskeletal dysfunction are normally functional and are generally related to muscle hypertonicity and joint blockage. Once a joint has lost the normal range of motion, the muscles surrounding the joint will reduce the stress on the area. A restriction in a joint can lead to muscle imbalance and postural distortions. Releasing a tight muscle will normally release joint restriction but you must have a complete understanding of how everything works as a unit.

Muscular dysfunction is not restricted to a local area. Dysfunction is an interrelationship between connective tissue and the nervous system. Anyone treating musculoskeletal dysfunction should possess a wide range of skills that can allow him/her to identify both joint and soft tissue restrictions or the end result will not be as good as it could be.

The normal response of a muscle to stress is to intensify the tonal quality. Increased stress on the soft tissue creates hypertonicity and pain. This type of stress on a muscle can cause postural imbalances, strain patterns, structural imbalance, repetitive strain, emotional strain, trauma and fibrosis, immobilization, and nutritional inefficiencies. Any combination of these factors can cause compensation, as a result of the increased muscle tone. The antagonist to a hypertonic muscle becomes weaker, waste product build-up, and oxygen deprivation can occur due to ischemia. Pain can occur from hypertonic muscles being stressed at the tendons and insertions. When the hypertonic structures cross a joint, imbalances can be a result of dysfunctional movement patterns.

You need to be educated so you are capable of treating pain and dysfunction and to be successful in your career. Knowing anatomy and the function of each of the body's systems is necessary in the decision of what type of bodywork is most appropriate. Understanding anatomy, kinesiology, and pathology can make your massage more precise, effective, and successful.

Points to remember when thinking about anatomy:

- Keep your memory up-to-date about anatomy and landmarks so you will always use superior palpation skills.
- Understand the role of each body part and how everything works together as a whole.
- Muscles pull the bones.
- Postural muscles uphold your posture and do not tire easily.
- Phasic muscles are more for movement and fatigue easily.
- Frequently educate yourself so that you can help reduce your client's pain and dysfunction.

Chapter Seven

Repetitive Strain and Overuse Injuries

Imagine the frustration, fear, and isolation that you would feel if you were injured and could not do the work you loved. Now, see yourself taking care of your body, working without injury, and always being able to do the work you love to do. The healthy, injury-free scenario is where you always want to be. If you are healthy, it is hard to imagine the physical pain and depressed feelings one has when an injury has occurred. A therapist that has an overuse injury does not always look injured and because the symptoms are multi-faceted it can be frustrating and confusing.

A repetitive strain injury (RSI) or an overuse injury is a cumulative trauma disorder stemming from prolonged repetitive, forceful, or awkward hand movements. In opposition to what people may think, the hands are not the only part of the body that can have a repetitive strain injury. Many parts of the body can be overused and injured. Repetitive strain or overuse syndrome is created from strain to a certain body part that can become chronic and includes a wide range of conditions. Some examples of overuse syndrome include: tendonitis, tenosynovitis, bursitis, nerve impingements such as carpal tunnel and thoracic outlet, shin splints, and various other musculoskeletal injuries.

Overuse injuries are generally an outcome of repetitive use, inefficient movement, poor or static posture, and stress to the soft tissues of the body. Connective tissue hardens over time because the soft tissue is overused. This is a natural response for the prevention of injury. Any repetitive action that places excessive strain on the soft tissues can cause damage to the body. Microscopic damage occurs in the soft tissue and can build up over time. The damage that develops can cause excessive strain, tearing, and inflammation. Injuries to the soft tissue are common and can include strains, sprains, tendonitis, and possible tearing. Injuries can happen when there is not proper healing time for the soft tissue to repair. This type of injury is commonly seen in muscles, tendons, and ligaments.

Injuries are classified as either acute (traumatic), or chronic (overuse). Acute injuries come from a specific impact or trauma and occur suddenly during an activity. Symptoms of an acute injury are severe pain, inability to bear weight on a limb, tenderness and weakness in a limb, and decreased range of motion. On the other hand, chronic injuries are normally a result of overusing a part of the body while engaged in a sport or exercise and happen over a long period of time. Symptoms of a chronic injury are swelling, pain when performing specific activities, decreased strength, reduced range of motion of the joint, muscle soreness, numbness, and a dull ache at rest.

The muscular system looks very complex; but, it is very simple. A muscle can do two things: either contract and relax or lengthen and shorten. The system is made of simple levers and pulleys. The whole muscular system works together to manage the stresses caused by gravity when movement takes place. The muscular system develops in accordance with the way we use, abuse, or overuse our bodies. Overuse develops in the parts of the body that are under the greatest stress or repetitive use, compared to other parts of the body.

Human muscles are designed for repetitive movements. In fact, muscles are fairly good at doing contractions repeatedly. What muscles are not designed for are static contractions. A static contraction happens when a muscle holds a position against an opposing force. When a muscle is held in this type of position it has to work very hard. A muscle held in static contraction also burns a lot of oxygen and carbohydrates for fuel and closes off its own blood supply, decreasing circulation and limiting admission of much needed fuel. Tight muscles can accumulate waste products and form fibrosis or knots in the muscles. With repetition and constant contraction, muscle fibrosis can accumulate over time and then pain can set in. When muscles are held in a fixed or tense position, circulation is decreased and the muscles become fatigued. In effect, blood vessels constrict from the muscles being tense and the nerves can become compressed. It may take years for this damage to build up and it can take a while to reverse this damage. The best way to deal with repetitive strain is to not let it happen in the first place.

The amount of strain a body can take before injury occurs depends on many factors. Poor technique and improper training can be a causative factor. Individual, biomechanical, and technical factors can all play a part in an injury. Age, diet, health, lifestyle, joint instability, and previous injuries all affect how easy an injury can occur. Finally, the strength, conditioning, and flexibility of an individual can also be factors in the injury process.

Strains, sprains, tendonitis, and tenosynovitis are among the injuries that can occur with repetitive stress. Muscles, tendons, and ligaments are arranged with parallel fibers and, when injured, some of the fibers can be torn. The injury severity depends on the amount of fibers torn. For example, first-degree injuries involve a few torn fibers, second-degree injury are worse with more fibers torn, and third-degree injuries are ruptures that can be disconnected from the bone.

Muscles contract and relax to help the body move in a variety of ways. When a muscle contracts it pulls on the tendon, which is connected to the bone. A strain can happen in a muscle or tendon that has been stretched too far, twisted, or torn. Muscle strains can occur when too much tension is placed on the muscle while it is in contraction, especially in the eccentric contraction phase. Most strains are minor. If a strain does not receive proper treatment and healing time, it can repair inadequately which can result in scarring and adhesions. Tears can happen anywhere along the muscle, especially at the muscle-tendon junction. Symptoms of a strain include swelling, bruising, pain at rest, and pain with movement. The muscle may be unable to move and it may spasm, depending on the severity.

Muscles learn bad habits or inefficient movement patterns from overuse. Splinting, guarding, and substitution can occur over time. Splinting is a contracting of the muscle to protect an area and guard against pain. Eventually, the muscles that are in spasm can lose their ability to relax and the state can become chronic. Muscles easily develop habits that are hard to break. Substitution of certain muscles can happen when an injury or overuse has taken place. When certain muscles do not move as they are meant to, other muscles will take over. When this occurs, the muscle that takes over has to do an additional job and sets this muscle up for overuse.

Two common areas for a muscle strain are the back and the hamstrings. Most strains are acute because muscles have good blood supply which aids in faster healing to the muscle. An overuse strain can develop slowly with repetitive motion. As a result, the symptoms build up slowly and can become chronic without even being in an acute stage. Chronic strains can occur in the muscle and tendon, consequently, because of the overuse and repetitive motion. Any movements that create pain are to be avoided until the pain has subsided. When the pain dissipates, movement can be added slowly and with moderation to build strength back.

Tendonitis is an injury and inflammation of the tendon usually at the musculotendinous junction. Tendons are more susceptible to strain if tension is applied too quickly or if the tendon is not warmed up properly. Other ways that a tendon could be strained is if the tendon is weak or the tendon or muscle is tense or contracted when force is applied. Tendonitis can happen anywhere along the tendon but is generally more common where the tissue composition changes. The symptoms of tendonitis are comparable to muscle strains, but sometimes are more intense. In the acute stage, some heat and swelling may be visible and resisted movements can cause pain. The healing of a tendon is slower than a muscle and depends on the subacute phase and scar tissue development. Stretching the area in the subacute stage assists the fibers to rearrange and realign. If the injured tendon has too little weight bearing with healing and does not regain flexibility, the tendon will be weak because of adhesion. The right amount of stretching, weight bearing, movement, and scar tissue alignment are crucial to healing an injured tendon.

Tenosynovitis is an inflammation of a tendon that passes through a synovial sheath. These sheaths are made of connective tissue and are lubricated with synovial fluid. Repetitive movement and stress in this type of area can cause the sheath to become inflamed. This condition can arise from local infection but mostly comes from some type of mechanical stress. Examples of symptoms in the acute phase include: local pain, heat, stiffness, and swelling. In the subacute phase, only pain and stiffness may be present. The tendon may feel or sound grainy as it moves through the sheath. Tenosynovitis is very common around the wrist. Tendinosis is an injury to a tendon that has been damaged significantly but is no longer inflamed. The injured tendon usually has misaligned scar tissue and loss of strength. Inflammation is involved in the initial stages of an injury. However, it is actually the incomplete healing that causes the pain and disability. Cross-fiber friction massage followed by ice massage can help to realign the fibers and heal an injured tendon.

Ligaments hold bone together and offer little pliability and stretch. A sprain refers to an injured ligament. A stressed ligament will usually tear before it stretches. If a ligament gets stretched, it will not spring back to its original length and it will not assist with stabilizing the joint. The laxity of the ligament can become chronic and the ligament can be re-injured easily. Sprains can sometimes be more serious than a strain because ligaments are less elastic and are slower to heal. Sprains also tend to swell rapidly to immobilize the joint. Acute sprains show inflammation with a loss of function. In the subacute phase, inflammation may still be present but the joint is more mobile. The joints most vulnerable to sprains are the ankle, knee, and wrist. Therapists can sprain the wrist with excessive deep tissue strokes using the fist and can sprain the fingers if used as a primary tool for stripping.

Common types of injuries most therapists deal with are in the muscle, tendon or ligament. Strains, sprains, and tendonitis respond well to massage in the subacute phase. The subacute phase is the best time to apply massage for realigning scar tissue because the injury is more recent. Cross-fiber, linear friction, and proprioceptive neuromuscular facilitation (PNF) are all helpful to heal injured tissue. The sooner an injury is treated, the better chance it has to heal completely without becoming chronic.

Another common result of overuse that often occurs with a bodyworker is arthritis. Your body includes one hundred and forty seven different joints. The main areas that could become arthritic are the joints of the hands, hips, spine, feet, and knees. Osteoarthritis creates progressive degeneration of the cartilage in the joint and is associated with wear and tear. Any damage done to the body can cause arthritis. Primary osteoarthritis is caused from a gradual degeneration of the joint through sports or heavy labor. Secondary osteoarthritis is from injury or repeated injury to a joint, mechanical imbalance, or some type of congenital problem. With this type of arthritis, the cartilage is gradually destroyed, the raw bone is unprotected, and the joint becomes very tender and can be extremely painful. This cartilage cannot be replaced and so the body repairs it with bone and can create bone spurs around the arthritic joint. Symptoms can include stiffness and crepitus in a joint, swelling and pain in the joint, synovitis, and visual signs of inflammation around the joint. Symptoms will start out intermittently and can be worse in the morning. Light exercise can help keep the joint mobile if the exercise does not apply too much pressure or stress the joint. Correcting muscle imbalance with proper exercise and stretching is helpful to reduce wear and tear on the joint and reduce pain.

Dysfunction in the musculoskeletal system can cause a disturbance in the peripheral nervous system and create nerve compression. The symptoms feel as if they originate in the local tissues, most of the time, the cause is along the path of the nerve. Numbness, tingling, and burning are symptoms of nerve disruption. The compression or entrapment can occur where the nerve passes through a moving joint structure. Nerve compression and entrapment happens, either when a bone or disk compresses a nerve, or can take place when soft tissue presses on a nerve.

Carpal tunnel syndrome (CTS) is a set of symptoms that occur from entrapment of the median nerve. Carpal tunnel syndrome can occur from overusing the muscles, thus creating inflammation within the tendons and nerves that pass through the tunnel. Carpal tunnel syndrome can cause pain, tingling, numbness, and weakness in the hand. The most common reason for carpal tunnel syndrome is the narrowing of the carpal tunnel. The carpal tunnel can decrease in size due to muscle tension or from the carpal ligament compressing above the tunnel. The reduction in space in the carpal tunnel also can be due to muscle imbalance between the flexors and extensors. The flexor muscles become shortened and thicker and the extensors become weak and are unable to hold the carpal bones in place. The tunnel can collapse in on itself and cause friction with the flexor tendons. This friction causes irritation and inflammation as well as, decreases space in the tunnel. The solution for eliminating muscle imbalance is to stretch and lengthen the flexors and stretch and strengthen the extensor muscles. Maintaining muscle balance is the key to stabilizing the carpal bones and preventing them from collapsing into the carpal tunnel. Edema is another common cause of carpal tunnel symptoms and causes added pressure in a space where there is no extra room. Edema caused from pregnancy, obesity, or menopause is common and usually bilateral. Essential steps to reducing nerve problems in the carpal tunnel area are to decrease the inflammation and rest the area completely. When the inflammation and symptoms have subsided, break up the scar tissue and release the flexor retinaculum. Massaging the muscles in the nerve related path could be effective in relieving the compression of the nerve. Receiving massage is indicated for carpal tunnel, but with caution. If any of the same symptoms become present when massage is applied to the hand and wrist, disregard the treatment immediately. Certain types of carpal tunnel respond well to massage. It is important that you confirm that a medical doctor has diagnosed the disorder and know the main cause of the symptoms before applying massage to make sure it is indicated.

Thoracic outlet syndrome (TOS) is a neurovascular entrapment and is common among therapists who have poor posture. Poor posture such as slumping and anteriorly rotating the shoulders can bring the clavicle close to the first rib and reduce the size of the thoracic outlet. Reducing this space entraps the nerves of the brachial plexus and can disrupt nerve impulse. In turn, this reduction in space can initiate loss of strength and create numbness and tingling from the thoracic outlet to the fingertips. In the early stage, discomfort can occur while doing massage. In the later stage, pain and discomfort becomes more prominent and frequent. Thoracic outlet can be caused from anything that impairs functioning of the brachial plexus. Some examples that can cause reduction in nerve impulse from the brachial plexus are subluxation of cervical vertebra, misalignment of the first rib, spondylosis, and atrophy of muscles. Signs and symptoms of thoracic outlet syndrome (TOS) are numbness, tingling, shooting pains moving to or from the arm, or a combination of both. Have orthopedic tests to determine the diagnosis. Pain in the shoulders, arms, and hands have many different reasons and can often be misdiagnosed because soft tissue injuries do not always show up on medical tests. Like carpal tunnel, the treatment for thoracic outlet depends entirely on what produced the symptoms. Resting of the affected area and reducing the entrapment is important to treating the condition. If the condition is related to tight muscles or muscle spasm, receiving massage to the scalenes and pectoralis minor is recommended. Also, specific stretches and exercises for the pectoralis minor, scalenes, and their antagonists can make a difference in the reoccurrence of symptoms.

Double crush syndrome is more commonly seen than people think and could be noticed with TOS and CTS. Cervical root compression can be found in combination with CTS. It only takes the weight of a nickel to compress a nerve. If the nerve is compressed with this small amount of pressure, it can impede the nerve flow by thirty percent. With nerve compression, a safety margin could be exceeded if you have a more proximal nerve lesion. Two minimal nerve compressions are more severe than a single compression. The diagnosis of double crush syndrome can be made only if the same nerve fiber is compressed at two different sites. In addition, the clinical manifestation of a double crush is caused from loss of nerve conduction. Examples are nerve dysfunctions such as sensory deficits or muscle weakness. Conservative treatment should be used initially and each entrapment needs to be located. Treatment should be conducted at each lesion for the best results. Double crush is still treated as a theory and challenged by medical professions but is a very real disease to the patients involved.

Myofascial pain is a widespread cause of pain today. The constant overloading of muscles on the job is common these days. Overusing and overloading the muscles can lead to myofascial pain. Trigger points can occur in the myofascia, skin, ligaments, and bone lining and can contribute to myofascial pain. A trigger point is a hyperirritable, localized spot in muscle or soft tissue that is palpable as a knot or rigid band that can cause local or referred pain. Trigger points can occur from overuse, injury, and fatigue of muscle tissue. Joint problems and surgery can also create trigger points in the tissue. Trigger points can entrap the nerves, blood, and lymph vessels and can cause a variety of confusing symptoms. Active trigger points produce pain locally or in a more remote location. Each particular trigger point has a referral pain pattern. An active trigger point hurts when the specific muscle is used and can continue to hurt even at rest. A latent trigger point exists but does not actively refer pain until the area is strained. A latent trigger point does not usually hurt unless it is pressed yet it can restrict movement, weaken, and shorten the affected muscle. Latent trigger points can be made active by overuse, overstretching, or chilling of a muscle. Central trigger points are located in the center of the muscle where the motor nerve is located and where tissue can get bound up. Treating trigger points and myofascial pain starts with locating the central point in the belly of the muscle, which is helpful for reducing referred pain.

Trigger points can be deactivated if treated correctly and perpetuating factors can be avoided. Trigger points that are left untreated or not treated thoroughly can still cause pain. Movement is sometimes restricted to avoid pain and the trigger point can become latent. If the muscle is still overworked without being treated, active trigger points can develop secondary and satellite trigger points. Secondary trigger points arise when a muscle is stressed because it has to take over the job of another muscle. Satellite trigger points can occur in the referred pain zone of another trigger point. Without proper treatment and deactivation of trigger points, widespread pain can develop.

Muscle strains, tendonitis, sprains, arthritis, nerve impingement syndromes, and myofascial pain are realities in the massage and bodywork field. Bodywork is a physical occupation and should be considered a sport itself. Most sessions are performed for an hour and a therapist may do up to eight hourly sessions a day. The upper body is subject to a lot of stress in this career. The arms are not exceptionally aerobic muscles and are prone to overuse since their movements are particularly intricate.

Think of yourself as a massage athlete. Performing massage is very strenuous on your hands and upper extremities. At some point in your career it is very likely that an injury could occur. This type of physical work demands skill, strength, and endurance, just like a track and field runner or baseball player. The part of the body used in a sport is the one most probable to become injured. A baseball player would be more inclined to injure the elbow, the rotator cuff, or the shoulder joint and a massage therapist would be most likely to injure the rotator cuff, the thumb, or the tendons in the forearm.

A competitive athlete in any sport trains often and knows that during each workout some damage is being done in the muscles and joints that are being used. The damage is accepted because the athlete knows if proper nutrition and rest are given the tissues will repair themselves in time for the next workout. A marathon runner runs 10 miles a day, 6 days per week. She eats well, stretches before and after every run, and sleeps 8 to 9 hours each night. She understands that running is hard on her body and knows that microscopic injuries are occurring in her legs and feet. She also knows that she lives in an amazing human body that can repair and rebuild itself while she sleeps. She eats a lot of vegetables, whole grains, chicken, and fish. She avoids sugar and white flour, consumes small amounts of alcohol and caffeine, and does not use nicotine. She understands that her body cannot repair with candy bars and soda pop. She realizes that running 10 miles per day requires a repair rate that must be faster than the damage rate. She repairs by supplying the muscles with a lot of fresh water, oxygen, and healthy food. She wears quality shoes and changes them often, runs on even surfaces, and stretches frequently. She is aware that increased flexibility helps to absorb the shock and the more flexibility she has the less damage that will be done with each day of training. The marathon runner knows her limit is 10 miles. She tried to run 12 miles and was in pain after a couple of weeks of running. During those few weeks, she did not get 8 hours of sleep at night and tried to make up for it with a couple of cups of coffee. Her lack of self-care caused her legs to hurt. Subsequently, she resumed her healthy habits and her legs no longer hurt. She found that if she wore the wrong shoes, did not get enough sleep, and did not stretch often it would result in pain.

A massage therapist has a lot in common with a marathon runner. A certain amount of damage occurs in the muscles every day, and every night a certain amount of repair takes place. If the amount of repair can equal that of damage, then the next day you can work at 100 percent. If you only repair at 99 percent you will feel fine, but if this occurs over time and you continue to repair at a deficiency, you will be on a downhill slide. Before you know it you will only be operating at 70 or 80 percent because you forgot to stretch one day, did not eat healthy, or had excessive stress. Fatigue will be your biggest telltale. You will come home tired and you will wake up tired. You are more achy than normal and soon it turns to pain. Driving, brushing your hair and teeth, and doing everyday functions starts to cause you pain. This can seem to happen suddenly, but it actually happens over time. It only takes a small difference between the repair and damage rate to create an injury. On the other hand, it only takes small measures to ensure longevity and prevent damage from occurring. A healthy body maintains a neutral balance between damage and repair. This neutral balance of staying healthy may be interrupted if the damage rate is slowed or if the damage rate occurs too rapid to be healed.

Overtraining in the massage field means that overload is occurring in the soft tissues and/or not enough recovery time is being allowed. The symptoms of overtraining are just like an athlete and include: fatigue, lack of energy, pain in the muscles and joints, irritability, insomnia, and depression. Rest, in the form of less activity or sleep, is essential for the treatment of overtraining. You can track your resting heart rate every morning to know if you are overtraining. If any rise in the heart rate is noted, you may not be fully recovered from the previous day. The most important barometer to know if you are overtraining is to be aware of your body. Pay attention to your mood and your mental state. Research has suggested that rest is the most effective way to treat overtraining, whether it is time off from the sport, work, or just some additional sleep.

Overuse injuries include slight or vague symptoms that develop gradually and these symptoms arise as subtle, aching pains and develop over time. Symptoms may get worse after a sudden burst of activity, increased workload, or unaccustomed movements. Eventually, these symptoms can grow into a devastating injury if not cared for and healed properly. The main factors of an overuse injury arise from using incorrect body mechanics, increasing workload too quickly, not allowing enough time for rest and recovery, overtraining, or returning from an injury too quickly.

Some injuries are very apparent. Even so, overuse injuries occur progressively over time and the damage that occurs from constant and repetitive straining of the body part is cumulative. Remodeling is an internal process that includes the breakdown and build-up of tissue. If breakdown happens faster than build-up, an injury can occur. Chronic, overuse injuries come about if you do not pay attention to the warning signs your body gives you. Warning signs can be subtle at the beginning of an overuse injury, but become more apparent when damage has occurred. Warning signs vary from person to person and from specific injury. Warning signs of an overuse injury could include: reduced range of motion, comparative weakness, joint pain, persistent pain in the area of repetitive use, swelling, tingling, or numbness. If you notice any of these warning signs, stop the activity you are doing. It is highly suggested to pay attention to these sensations at the first sign, in the initial phase. The main goals are to prevent further damage, find the source of injury, and begin treatment immediately.

A repetitive injury can turn into a syndrome if not cared for properly. Repetitive strain injury (RSI) can also be called overuse syndrome, cumulative trauma disorder, or occupational overuse syndrome. This condition results from overuse of a part of your body or an activity that involves repetitive movement. Overuse syndrome occurs when a group of muscles are used repeatedly without adequate rest. Repeating a movement over and over can create tightness and overuse in one muscle group while the opposing muscle group becomes weak and underused. Repetitive stress on the tissues can cause a muscle or tendon to be overstretched, a muscle or tendon to be shortened from constant contraction, joints and tendons to be overloaded, or nerve impingement. Overuse causes hypoxia, possible muscle spasms, and microtearing in the tissue. If the area is not allowed to heal, the effects can be cumulative and an overuse injury can take place.

The terms, repetitive use injury and repetitive use syndrome, are used concurrently, although the term syndrome can be used with a more serious or chronic condition. Repetitive use injuries have different levels that range from a grade one to a grade five. In a grade one overuse injury, pain is only present when performing work and daily activities. With a grade two overuse syndrome, pain subsides by evening and daily activities are mildly affected. Pain and tenderness are only mild. Therapists with grades one and two can still normally work with some modifications. With a grade three overuse injury; pain continues into the evening but is not present upon waking. Signs of pain are evident a short time after you begin working and daily living is affected. Grade three requires an absence from work. You can return to work, depending on recovery time and job modifications. It is a good idea to take time off until the symptoms dissipate completely. With a grade four overuse injury, pain upon waking is present during each working day and at night. Symptoms can subside on weekend or days off; but, if you want the injury to heal and not repeat itself, let the symptoms dissipate completely. People with grade four injuries infrequently return to the same working position unless they are off for months. Finally, with a grade five injury, pain is ongoing and daily life is completely restricted. People with a grade five, overuse syndrome rarely return to their line of work or to the job force at all. Physical symptoms that occur with each grade and severity consist of tenderness, swelling, numbness, redness, spasms, tingling, burning, and numbness.

Repetitive strain injuries (RSI) are complex for the medical professional, as well as the patient. Symptoms are different for each person and the recovery process and time frame can be unique to each person. Advice from each professional can be contradictory and the process can get very frustrating, particularly if you cannot continue to work until the injury is fully healed. Contact a specialist and find the root cause of the symptom(s). A repetitive strain injury is biomechanical and muscle imbalances needs to be addressed. A quick-fix solution will not usually work since it takes time, patience, and perseverance to restore proper functioning to a body that has been misused over time.

Returning to work after an injury depends on the individual because each injury is unique. Make sure your doctor has cleared you before returning to work. Going back to work too soon can cause re-injury and can develop into a chronic problem. Guidelines for a safe return to work include: being pain-free, having full range of motion, being full or close to full strength, no visible edema, and all symptoms must have subsided. Proper conditioning of your body before an injury occurs can help you to recover more rapidly. Always follow your doctor's advice when returning to work and treat your injuries as soon as symptoms appear.

Massage therapists think of themselves more as caregivers and not of the physical work they are doing. Just like an athlete, you need to exercise, stretch, and take time off when injured to heal. Injuries do occur. When an injury does happen, do not feel ashamed and realize you are an athlete that may need to rest and to take time off from doing what caused the injury in the first place. Time off is invaluable for an injury to heal completely and is essential for the prevention of a chronic condition.

Points to remember so you can avoid a repetitive stress injury:

- Have good posture and body mechanics.
- Be aware of the tension in your body.
- If it hurts, stop!
- Cover your hands and keep them from getting chilled when sleeping.
- Make sure your palms face your body instead of your thumbs while sleeping.
- Exercise to increase circulation.
- Ice your hands to remove inflammation.
- Get proper treatment and medical support from a Medical doctor, chiropractor, massage therapist, and acupuncturist.
- Avoid other hand intensive activities to reduce strain.
- Takes frequent breaks to rest and recover.
- Be proactive and responsible for your own health.

Chapter Eight

My Story

I have been in the massage therapy profession for over ten years. I really enjoy the physical component of my job and the satisfaction I receive from helping people to relax, heal, and rejuvenate. I have had a very abundant professional career and have worked in many facets of this profession. I worked for myself and for large corporations, and I also have worked in the educational aspect of massage. The spa that I worked at, on the strip, in Las Vegas was a great place for me to grow professionally. At this place of employment, I was taught a lot about professionalism and I learned many great treatments and massage modalities.

A unique type of massage I did at this spa was barefoot deep compression massage. The results I noticed for the clients were substantial after doing a barefoot massage. Since this type of massage is performed with oil, the therapist can glide on the client's skin and lengthen the connective tissue. The fascia is lengthened and the disc space is increased in the client. I really enjoyed this modality and had fun performing it.

This type of massage is like a dance and uses the body in a different way than regular massage with the hands. Conventional massage uses the hands as the main instrument, whereas barefoot massage uses the feet to deliver the pressure. Massage, using the hands, applies power generated from the feet pushing off the ground and then transfers power through to the hands. With barefoot massage, the arms and hands are used to apply oil and to hold onto the bars overhead for balance. Power is generated from the core and is transferred to the legs and through the feet. The feet are used as the hands in this type of massage. This is an extremely effective type of massage for the client and the therapist gets to use their body in a different way. Barefoot massage is a good massage for using broad and general strokes on the client's body, especially the back and larger muscles of the legs.

In addition to doing other styles of massage, I performed many of the barefoot massages. I received massage therapy on my upper body, but not as much on the lower body. I stretched my whole body but, after a while, my legs still felt tight. I kept in shape by doing yoga and cardiovascular exercise on the bike, elliptical machine, and the treadmill. I felt that I needed to be in shape to perform this massage even though it could have contributed to the tightening of the connective tissue. I noticed that the fascia was progressively getting tighter on the plantar surface of my feet, two months prior to the injury. I released the trigger points in my lower legs and feet and the fascia felt looser. The constriction felt better for a month but it came back accompanied with burning around the medial ankles. I notified a manager and they said to let them know if I wanted to be taken off the book for this massage. This treatment was my favorite and I was not willing to stop doing what was causing the discomfort. So, I continued doing barefoot massage; even though I knew better. A month later, the muscles, tendons and fascia constricted further and as a result, the pain in each heel and burning of the medial ankles worsened. A few days later, I could not walk because of the hypertonicity in the soft tissue. I went to a chiropractor and took a few days off. The chiropractor did muscle and laser therapy and diagnosed my problem as Plantar Fasciitis.

I returned to work and notified my employer of the injury. I was sent to a workers compensation clinic and was diagnosed with Achilles Tendonitis and Plantar Fasciitis. I returned to work on light duty with certain job restrictions and I was to perform only Swedish massage with my hands and no barefoot massage. After a few weeks of light duty, the burning increased and tingling started in each medial ankle and foot because I was still on my feet doing massage and walking throughout the large spa. I continued working on light duty, which amounted to three massages a day. This light duty situation continued for nine weeks. I applied ice to my feet and took an anti-inflammatory medication but things only got worse. The tingling and burning in my feet persisted because I was not allowed enough rest time to heal.

Finally, I was referred to an orthopedic specialist by workers compensation. This doctor did not examine or even touch my feet. I told him that my feet were tingling and numb. He told me he would not take me off of work and that he had no quick answers for me. I left his office feeling very frustrated. When I was notified of the next doctor's appointment, I was apprehensive. I decided to be open-minded and positive about this doctor. He was a podiatric surgeon and was very knowledgeable and cordial. He diagnosed me with bilateral Achilles Tendonitis and Overuse Syndrome. The doctor strapped my feet in an attempt to lessen the symptoms and ordered orthotics to correct the overpronation in my feet. The tingling and burning sensations continued and the doctor took me off work completely so I could heal. Six weeks later I had an MRI on both feet and ankles. The MRI reported edema in both of my ankle joints, bilateral subtalar synovitis, and edema in the sheath of the posterior tibial tendons. The doctor said the inflammation was from repetitive use and not from a specific trauma. He also diagnosed the tingling and burning sensations under the medial malleoli as tarsal tunnel syndrome. The doctor decided to give me a cortisone shot in each subtalar joint. When he injected the medication, I felt a referral into the tarsal tunnel. The pain in this area lessened after a few days. The next week, the doctor gave me another cortisone shot in both ankle joints. The after effects of this shot were very difficult and for three days it was very painful to walk and so I crawled around my house. The pain did lessen after a few days but the ankles were still sore to walk on.

The doctor believed the main reason for the tarsal tunnel symptoms was from the inflammation pressing on the nerves and scar tissue impeding the nerve flow. The cortisone did help the tarsal tunnel pain medially but I could still feel tingling on the top of the left foot and into the toes. This was diagnosed as anterior tarsal tunnel. The ankles continued to feel very sore when I walked and especially when I stood in one place. I had to start walking with a cane because of the pain, accompanied by muscle atrophy and weakness. The tarsal tunnel pressure, pain, and numbness returned and the second cortisone shot in the subtalar joint was painful and not effective.

The doctor treated me conservatively since the nature of the injury was from overuse. He explained to me that, with an overuse injury, it took many months and maybe even years for the damage to occur. It would take time to repair the damage done. The doctor approved swimming as an exercise. I was excited because I missed doing my cardiovascular exercise and since this exercise was non-weight bearing, it was a good alternative. I swam for six weeks but had to stop, given that my feet were more tingly and numb after the exercise. Rest and minimal use of the feet were recommended for healing. More information was needed, so the podiatrist sent me to different specialists with my own insurance. My doctor wanted to rule out lumbar radiculopathy as a source of the tingling and numbness in the feet.

Quite a few weeks later, I was sent to have nerve conduction and EMG tests performed on my legs and feet by workers compensation. The technician told me that there was some abnormality in the tarsal tunnel but the reports from the neurologist came back normal. The nerve conduction test aggravated the tarsal tunnel symptoms and the burning, tingling, and pain increased again. I went to another neurologist with my own insurance and he told me that I had classic symptoms of Multiple Sclerosis because of my antalgic gait. Luckily, my brain scans and blood work showed normal so Multiple Sclerosis was ruled out. I had MRIs of my brain, cervical, thoracic, and lumbar spine. In the lumbar spine the results showed annual fiber tears and prolapsed discs in L4-L5 and L5-S1. My chiropractor and the podiatrist both pointed out that they thought the nerve related symptoms in my feet were coming from the disc problems in my low back. I felt that the first nerve conduction tests were contradictory and I wanted another opinion so I went back to the previous neurologist. The neurologist repeated the nerve conduction tests and they came back normal. I was so upset. I knew what I felt in my feet was real especially since I lived with it on a daily basis. Why were the conduction tests showing normal?

I went to two neurosurgeons, one that workers compensation sent me to and the other I saw with my own insurance. I wanted an honest opinion and a solution, instead, I felt more frustrated then when I first walked into their offices. Even though I had disc pathology, I did not have major pain in my back or much radiation of pain down my legs. Consequently, neither of the neurosurgeons thought the symptoms in my feet were coming from my back. I was in denial that the symptoms were coming from my back because the pain and tingling were so intense in my feet. However, when I found out about the prolapsed discs, I did extensive research. I found a lot of interesting information as I continued on a quest to find answers, so I decided to write a medical paper on my condition with my treating doctor.

I found that tarsal tunnel is a compression neuropathy and because of the varying etiology and symptomatology, diagnosis and treatment can be difficult. Symptoms can range from aching pain to a burning and tingling sensation. Other symptoms of tarsal tunnel are pain from prolonged standing, loss of sensation from the ankles to the toes, electric shock sensations, gait abnormality, swelling of the feet, and sensory disturbance. Causative factors of this condition could be overpronation, tumors or cysts, arthritis, diabetes, repeated ankle sprain, trauma, and repetitive stress. Anything that puts excessive pressure or strain in the tarsal tunnel area can create tarsal tunnel syndrome. Tarsal tunnel syndrome can be more common in active individuals, athletes, and people who stand a lot.

Some doctors believe that nerve conduction tests are not the most reliable tests to rule out carpal tunnel or tarsal tunnel. Some research states that nerve conduction tests can be normal in patients that have tarsal tunnel syndrome and it is possible for one to have tarsal tunnel with normal results on nerve conduction tests. An alternate test, with a Pressure Specified Sensory Device allows the doctor to determine the level of nerve entrapment and has a lower false negative rate than electrodiagnostic tests, which could have false negative responses in 50 percent of the cases. Electrodiagnostic testing can also be more disappointing, expensive, and painful for the client.

The research I did revealed that a double crush syndrome could occur not only in the upper extremities, but in the lower extremities as well. Upton and McComas did research and coined the term double crush. A double crush happens when dysfunction to a nerve at one site lessens the functioning of the nerve cells and the nerve become more vulnerable to trauma in other locations.

Basically, it has to do with a multilevel nerve lesion and the presence of a proximal lesion causes distal areas of the nerve to become more vulnerable to compression. I had some minimal nerve compression from the prolapsed discs in my low back and when impingement occurred in the tarsal tunnel area from inflammation and scar tissue, the nerve exceeded the safety margin and the symptoms were noticed distally. The research I found from Upton and McComas mentioned that 75 percent of the time, people with a proximal nerve root lesion close to the spine could have symptoms that arise in a more distal area. Most of the research done on double crush theory is on carpal tunnel and notes that two minimal nerve lesions or entrapments are more severe than one major entrapment. When a double crush is found, both crushes need to be treated for each area to be healed and the results of treatment to be successful.

The information on double crush theory was mostly on carpal tunnel and lesions in the cervical spine. I did find some information on lower extremity double crush but it was challenging and the information was on diabetic patients. I found that one of the most unnoticed factors in tarsal tunnel could be one of a double crush. Prolapsed discs pressing on L5 and/or S1 nerve roots could suggest a double crush syndrome where one crush or nerve impingement is in the low back and the second is in the tarsal tunnel area.

Since both impingements have to be addressed to treat double crush syndrome, it was time to treat the first impingement at the discs of L4-L5 and L5-S1. After three treatments on the DRX-9000tm spinal decompression machine, I knew that the discs had something to do with the symptoms in my feet. The DRX-9000tm is a machine that decompresses the spine and places a load on a specific disc to help relieve the neurocompression. When I was on the machine getting treatment I could feel the nerves waking up and a tingling sensation in my feet. This machine helped my symptoms and treated the disc by relieving pressure and allowing the disc to move back into position and heal. I exceeded the therapeutic dose of 32 treatments and the tingling was still present but it was definitely more manageable.

After 11 months, I still wanted more explanation, so I went to see an orthopedic surgeon. He was very pleasant and explained to me that he thought some of the symptoms were from my back and that the compression had caused the nerves to become chronically irritated and inflamed. He also thought arthroscopic surgery on the subtalar joint could bring me some relief. I saw another orthopedic surgeon in New Jersey to get his opinion. He said I definitely had lumbar radiculopathy that made my feet feel tingly and numb. This doctor told me that my fifth lumbar vertebra was fused on the left side to the sacrum, which was called Bertolotti's syndrome. This syndrome was not the cause of my problem but it contributed because degenerative disc disease is more likely with this syndrome. This transitional vertebra articulates with the sacrum and accelerates degeneration of the fourth lumbar disc. This results in limited movement at the lumbo-sacral connection and is compensated for in the upper segments. I did have a congenital malformation but nevertheless, performing deep barefoot compression massage caused excessive strain to the lower lumbar discs which resulted in the annular fiber tears.

The lower lumbar discs had annular fiber tears which leaked fluid out and irritated the nerves. There was compression on the discs but it was a matter of chemical irritation to the nerve, in addition to mechanical compression. This made sense to me because, after the therapeutic dose on the DRX-9000tm, the symptoms should have completely ceased. The DRX-9000tm is one of the most valuable treatments in healing the discs and taking pressure off the nerve. Now, I had to get treatment to reduce the inflammation of the nerve exiting the spine. I had to be patient and realize that nerves take a long time to heal, sometimes months or possible even years.

I went to a pain management doctor and received three epidural cortisone shots in my fourth and fifth discs and the facet joints to reduce the nerve inflammation. I had a 50 percent reduction in the tingling and the radicular pain down my left leg felt better. I decided that I would not do a discogram because it is invasive and could cause discitis. I already had enough problems and knew how to manage the pain and symptoms in my low back. I knew what worked for me so I continued with the treatments on the DRX-9000tm and used my inversion table whenever possible. I was lucky to have an excellent chiropractor that cared about my health and wanted to see me get better.

In the meantime, workers compensation insurance sent me to Los Angeles for an independent medical exam. They did not understand why I was not getting better and said my treating doctor was using me as an experiment. This was simply not true. The insurance company turned down every treatment my treating doctor ordered, so how was I supposed to get better? My situation was complicated but we had already figured it out. I had a double crush syndrome with two concurrent injuries. I did think that this orthopedic doctor in Los Angeles could offer some insight. Boy was I wrong. When workers compensation sends you to a doctor, most of the time, he is on their payroll and it shows. I knew the moment he started talking, he was not concerned about helping me. He asked me questions about how many massages that I performed and what I did on a daily basis. He looked at my ankle MRIs and said virtually nothing was wrong with my ankles. When I tried to show him the paper MRI report in my hand he would not look at it. He watched me walk and asked me to run. Was he crazy? It hurt so bad to even walk that there was no way I could run. He asked me what kind of job I could get in Las Vegas. I said that I did not know. I wanted to be fixed so I could work again. He said he could not tell me what was wrong and that I should go back to Las Vegas and find a job. I mentioned that some of the symptoms in my feet could be coming from my back. He said that was possible and that I should find a good rheumatologist and neurosurgeon when I got home. I felt so let down when I left. Tears streamed down my face as I flew back to Las Vegas and I wondered why this was happening to me. When I received the L.A. doctor's report it was a complete slap in the face. He said it was a non-industrial injury about twenty times and that he felt that I would have a full-blown rheumatologic condition someday. Six weeks later I received a letter from workers compensation stating that they were closing my case due to the nature of the non-industrial injury. Workers compensation gave me a final check for three days after I received the letter. I felt so betrayed and scared. I could not work because I was not better and I could not walk, must lest stand. Now, I had no income and wondered what I would do. Luckily, I have an amazing boyfriend and he told me not to worry because he would make sure everything was taken care of.

When I walked it hurt, especially when I walked on uneven surfaces. It literally brought tears to my eyes sometimes when I walked very far. I found out that because the doctor in Los Angeles said it was a "non-industrial" injury my private insurance would pay for the surgery. The universe does work in mysterious ways sometimes. I had put my full faith into just being well again. I did not care about the measly amount of money that I could have received from workers compensation. Sure it would have helped out but all I wanted to do was walk without pain. Since the conservative treatment was not reducing the symptoms, my treating doctor decided he would proceed with the arthroscopic surgery on both of my ankles. Finally, I was going to get the treatment I deserved and I would get better!

My treating doctor did arthroscopic surgery on the left subtalar and ankle joint in addition to a gastrocnemius recession, which is a lengthening of the gastrocnemius tendon. He found major adhesions in the subtalar joint and the ankle joint. The subtalar joint was fused with adhesions and caused the ankle joint to do the movement of both joints. This caused more inflammation and adhesion in the ankle joint. The adhesion and inflammation was creating pressure in the tarsal tunnel and creating tingling sensations in the tarsal tunnel area and into the big toe. No wonder it hurt to walk. The positive finding was that my cartilage was still healthy in these joints.

The surgery was harder on me than I thought it would be. There was a lot of trauma due to all the clean-up that had to be done. Both sides of my ankle were black and blue and very swollen. After three weeks, I was in a walking cast and was getting used to mobilizing with crutches. I began physical therapy the fourth week after surgery. My physical therapist was able to get more range of motion in the ankle and subtalar joints. It was still difficult to walk at this time because the fascia was very constricted around the area of the gastocnemius recession. The next week she used an e-stimulation machine that directly stimulated my peroneal nerve. This direct stimulation assisted movement of the joint and freed up some of the connective tissue. The next day, I massaged my legs and was able to walk. This made me happy. My physical therapist just had to get me to walk correctly. My gait was very dysfunctional because my movement patterns were off for over a year.

I went ahead with the surgery on my right foot six weeks after my left ankle. It was not as extensive as my left foot. However, the doctor still found a lot of adhesion in the subtalar joint and it was quite similar to the left foot. The adhesions were definitely from the unnatural foot motion I used while performing barefoot massage. When I got home from the hospital, I could not use my left foot to walk in to the house. The physical therapist had worked with me and I was bearing weight on the left foot but I did not realize that the neuromuscular pathway had been lost to my left foot. In addition, I did not realize I had lost the strength and balance on my left leg since I had not walked on it in six weeks. I was also disoriented and dizzy from anesthesia so I decided to crab walk into the house. I made it into the house pretty quickly and this was not the first time I had to crawl, so it was not a big deal. It was hard just to get to the bathroom. Luckily, the wheelchair was delivered a few hours later, which made it much easier to get around. It was harder to get around than I thought it would be. I should have waited a few more weeks to have the second surgery but I was anxious to get better. If there is a will then there is a way. The first four weeks were tough. I had to surrender to the situation and just stay down for three weeks. I wanted my left foot to be healed and to gain strength. I was determined and, as each day went on, I got better with bearing weight on my left foot and using my crutches. I knew all the pain would be worth it because I was finally going to better.

After a year and a half, I was on my two feet again. I had to relearn how to walk since I literally forgot how to walk correctly. I realized that I had a lot of pelvic instability from waddling and walking with an antalgic gait for so long. I had a lot of proprioceptive and muscular building to do. It was all worth it because I no longer walked with pain. My back definitely need more rehabilitation time but the symptoms were feeling better. I was walking better and I did not have to propel through my hips and upper body. After extensive physical therapy and a lot of healing time, I was better. All I had to live with was some numbness on the top of my left foot. I had to keep the compression off of my discs to reduce the radicular pain down my legs. I could definitely live with this because it did not interfere with my life. I could live a normal life now and did not to think about the pain with every step I took. I was so grateful. I just knew I would be happy and healthy in the end!

I did therapy consisting of Microvas(tm) (electrical stimulation for the muscles and nerves), acupuncture, DRX-9000(tm) spinal decompression therapy, epidural cortisone injections, cranial sacral therapy, Class IV low-level laser therapy, Reiki, structural integration, physical therapy, neuromuscular and deep tissue massage. All the treatments were valuable especially when used in conjunction with each other. I feel acupuncture and microvas(tm) helped to supply transmission to the nerves and prevent further nerve damage. All the other therapies helped my body to clear out waste products, increase blood supply and nutrients to the injured tissue, and realign connective tissue. Everything worked together to restore energy flow and support my body in self-correction and healing. Rest of the affected area was pertinent to reduce inflammation. Once inflammation subsided, it was time for rehabilitation and strengthening. I always had faith that things would eventually get better, but it was hard not being able to live a normal life. Some days were okay and some days were bad. Depression would happen at times but I would try to put myself back into a positive place and believe that things would improve.

The toll an injury takes physically, as well as mentally, on a person can be challenging. For me, depression occurred first, as a result of the pain, next from the isolation, and finally from the realization of how long and difficult my recovery was going to be. I went from being a very physical person to barely being able to walk into the next room. I was such an active person and this injury seemed to have taken my freedom away. I could not even go to the grocery store due to the pain and tingling in both feet. It was hard for me to live a normal life as a result of my restrictions. I could not do what I normally could so I would get so frustrated. I felt very vulnerable and weak. I also felt a loss of identity because I was isolated at home and could not do what I loved to do, which was to perform massage. When I became down or depressed, I tried to pull myself out of that state and think about what I was grateful for, however hard it was. Everyday I would focus on things I was thankful for even though it was easy to think of negative things. Constant monitoring of my thoughts and visualizing myself healed was necessary for my recovery.

I tried to be positive and make the best of my healing time. I read a lot and educated myself about different subjects. I explored my creativity with cooking while I was seated on a stool. I could still exercise as long as it was not weight bearing. I could do modified, seated yoga, core strengthening on a large exercise ball, weight and resistance training for my upper body, leg lifts, ball rolling, and Pilates. I did not want to let my body go and tried to be as active as I could.

Time, persistence, an excellent doctor, and proper rehabilitation were keys to my healing. My ankles did eventually heal, although it was a long, hard road to get there. There were some minor damages left over from the injury and I had to be careful not to overdue things with my legs and feet. With a repetitive use injury, the damage is cumulative and builds up over time. I know I should have paid more attention to the warning signs and stopped when I felt the tingling and burning sensations. Damage has already been done when these types of sensations show up. I will never be able to perform barefoot massage again. If I were to perform the same movements that caused the damage I would put myself at a higher risk for reinjury, especially since I had a grade five repetitive use injury.

It was hard for me to stand for hours in one place and to push off my feet to apply deep pressure so performing regular massage at a spa pace was no longer an option for me.

No two people will go through the same kind of healing nor will those people respond the same way to certain treatments. You have to learn what works best for you. You also have to take responsibility for your own health. You can sit around and wait for people to make you better, but that may never happen. This injury taught me that I had the ability to survive and I got to know myself on a deeper level. Also, I knew I could help others with an injury and the accompanying frustration, fear, and depression. I felt that I could be a source of inspiration and information for them.

The healing process was long. I put up with a long time of pain, burning, tingling, and numbness in my feet and went through many months of physical therapy. Finally, after a year and a half, I was on my feet again. I have returned to massage therapy but I only do massage with my hands on a few clients a week. I still use my skills with various energy modalities that allow my body to sit and I use my body with minimal intensity. Massage is my passion and, for that reason, I decided not to work at the arduous, physical pace I did before. I will be able to do massage for many more years because I am able to reduce the intensity on my body and perform massages and modalities that are less demanding.

This story should be a reminder to you that an injury can happen to anyone. My story should remind employers to do what is best for their employees, even if the employee thinks that he/she knows what is best for them. It is also pertinent for you as a therapist to stop an activity when sensations of tingling, burning, or numbness are present. Think of my feet as your hands. Pay attention to the cues your body gives you and take time off, when needed, to take care of yourself!

I cannot advise you on how to deal with workers compensation because I am not a lawyer and laws differ from state to state. I can tell you my experience with this system in hopes that it will inform you and lessen your frustrations. First, I made sure that I filed a report of injury with my employer. Notifying the employer of an injury is an important step; make sure it is filed and hopefully the case is accepted. Second, I asked if I had the right to choose my own medical provider. Third, I kept a pain diary and knew it was my right to get any of the doctor's notes and documentation. I also kept records of all phone calls I made or received and documented pertinent information concerning doctor appointment and therapies.

I held on to all the original paperwork I could and had a notebook of all the important phone numbers. I wrote down all the names of people I would talk to on the phone. I got calls from workers compensation nurses, but I knew I did not have to talk to them. Telling the nurses too much can lead to misinterpretations or misunderstandings. I had legal counsel because I knew this system would take advantage of my rights if I did not know what my rights were. I wrote down any questions I would have for my doctor so that I would not forget. When I was on light duty, I made sure the doctor was as specific as possible on my restrictions. These precise restrictions will help give the injured part time to heal. My symptoms got worse with light duty so I went to see a lawyer about my rights. I went to my family doctor to get documentation until I was able to see a specialist. I realized I was entitled to a second opinion if I was not satisfied with a doctor's diagnosis or recommendation. I read all of the letters I received from workers compensation and my lawyer would reply within the time allowed on the letter, if needed. Physical therapy can be very important to build strength and rehabilitate. Sometimes the system is willing to cover this type of therapy and sometimes they will not. I knew I was entitled to all of my medical files and I made sure I always got copies for myself. I made sure I thought about what I said because everything I said went into the notes. I learned that documentation is crucial and knowledge is power. Finally, I did not give up and I took control of my own health, which are the keys to surviving when involved in this type of situation. I also learned that some battles are worth fighting and some are not. Sometimes life is not fair and justice should be served but sometimes it cannot be. Do not give up on yourself because if you do then no one else can help you!

Notes

Chapter Nine

The Injury Process

You must understand that all injuries are not the same and healing time is as individual as each person is. Utilizing proper mechanics and leverage can reduce the risk of injury. Nevertheless, massage includes many repetitive movements and places a lot of stress on the joints, tendons, and ligaments. The body is not designed to do these kinds of stressful movements over an extended length of time and unfortunately injury can occur. An injury is likely to happen when the body is stressed past its normal limits.

Repetitive stress injuries (RSI) such as carpal tunnel or thoracic outlet are very common injuries for the massage therapist and bodyworker. Many other areas of the body are prone to injury in this profession as well. The neck and shoulders can be a common place of injury resulting from the shoulders being rotated internally, from the table height being too high, or from applying pressure from the strength of the upper extremities only. In this career, the wrists, hands, fingers, and thumbs are very vulnerable because of the constant strain that is used to perform massage. The knees are prone to injury when they are held in a locked position and when they are twisted while applying pressure. Furthermore, the low back is a common site of injury and can become injured from bending over too much from the waist, overarching when applying a stroke, or twisting while applying pressure. Muscles, joints, tendons, and nerves can be injured in this field and take time to heal once damage has occurred.

When tissues are injured, the body will automatically start to regenerate and repair. The healing process of an injury occurs in three phases. In phase one inflammation occurs, phase two includes tissue regeneration, and in phase three remodeling of the tissues take place. In phase one, the stage is set for repair. Phase one is the acute phase and occurs from the time of injury up until 72 hours after. Inflammation takes place and macrophages help to ingest debris as fibroblasts start to lay down the collagen fibers. Inflammation is a defense mechanism for the body and includes redness, swelling, heat, and pain. Swelling restricts circulation and applying ice at this time is very beneficial because it will help to reduce pain and swelling. It is important to understand that if inflammation did not take place, healing would not occur. This sets the stage for the first fibrils to be laid down to start the healing process.

The second phase of healing is called the proliferation or subacute phase. Many new blood vessels and capillaries are formed and they bring blood and oxygen to the area. Fibroblasts build up the area and collagen fibers pull the tissues back together. This phase takes place two to three days after the injury and can last up until six weeks later. The third phase of healing can also be called the remodeling phase and can start six weeks after the injury. This phase can last up to or over a year just depending on the severity of the injury. This phase can become a chronic phase of repair and can overlap with the subacute phase. During this phase, most inflammation has subsided but loss of function is likely. Pain can occur from stress to the area due to scar tissue formation. Scar tissue will strengthen as time passes; however, it will only be 70 to 80 percent as strong as the tissue it has replaced. During this last phase, you should be aware that avoidance of painful movements could become a habit. When movement is restricted, the remodeling and repair of tissues do not occur as completely. Also, normal function is not fully restored and symptoms persist if movement is completely avoided at this stage. When appropriate in this stage, regular exercise should be added to challenge the tissues so remodeling takes place. Exercises that are suitable for this phase have practical application and resistance should be added with body weight, elastic bands, and weights. The exercises should be shown by a professional and progressed slowly.

Of all the cells in the body, fibroblasts are the only cells we retain throughout our lives. Fibroblasts have a distinct property of being able to migrate to any part of the body. They regulate their internal chemistry according to local conditions and begin manufacturing specific structural tissue, appropriate to that area. No other cells demonstrate the extensive regenerative capabilities of fibroblasts. This makes them a key component in healing. Scar tissue is new collagen, made from fibroblasts that have migrated to the injury site.

The collagen fibers have been laid down and organized. At this time it is helpful to keep the collagen fibers from adhering to the surrounding tissues. The adhered fibers can be realigned in many ways. Some examples of realignment include: doing passive and active movements, keeping the site of injury mobile, and receiving massage therapy. If the scar or injury is left immobile for an extended amount of time, realignment of the tissue can be harder and re-injury could be more likely.

Most therapists believe that once pain has subsided, healing is complete. Even though inflammation and pain may have subsided, the actual healing process can take many weeks to completely heal. The period of healing after pain has decreased is the time when most re-injury occurs. Unfortunately, re-injury to a healed area is generally worse than the original injury because the tissue structure was already weak. The injury/re-injury cycle happens a lot with a massage therapist. Time and rest are essential to the healing process because an adequate amount of scar tissue has to form for stability. The period of time taken to rest the area is also important for healing and allows the inflammation to dissipate. If you re-injure the area by doing the same movement over and over, you will cause more inflammation and more scar tissue development. The cycle will continue and develop into a chronic state unless you rest and allow the inflammation to disperse.

If the cycle of injury or re-injury occurs you can be certain that muscle imbalance is involved. A part of the body can be either overdeveloped or not strong enough. Correcting and maintaining muscle balance between the agonist and antagonist muscle groups is crucial to maintaining health in your career. Lengthening and strengthening muscles that are subjected to overuse is quite important to preventing potential injury or rehabilitating existing injury.

Learn to recognize your body's signs of injury. The five signs of an injury include: swelling, heat, redness, pain, and loss of movement. Pain is the biggest sign that something is wrong. You should make a distinction of whether the pain is normal body use or one of injury. Usually, pain that is intermittent is something to pay attention to and may call for a decrease in workload, but pain that is constant is definitely a sign of injury and should be checked out by a doctor.

Pain is described as an unpleasant sensory or emotional experience related to actual or potential tissue damage. Pain is a feeling that is triggered in the nervous system. As a part of the body's defense system, pain is an important component of the body's ability to react to damaging stimuli. It is an early warning system to minimize injury. An injury triggers chemical reactions within pain sensors.

Electrical signals fire into the nervous system and travel to the brain. Nerves that sense pain work more slowly than others; a dull, throbbing pain operates so slowly that we sense a delay between the injury happening and the pain it triggers. This delay gives you time to free yourself from the cause of pain. Pain is processed in many parts of the brain. Pain is perception; it is the brain's interpretation of an injury. This is the reason why pain is different among various people. One person can look at a piece of art and see something totally different from another; this is because of perception. Pain has an emotional factor related to the experience and this emotional component colors the way a person perceives pain. For that reason, we all feel pain differently.

Pain may be sharp or dull and may come and go, or it may be constant. Pain is a helpful mechanism because, without pain, you could hurt yourself seriously without knowing it. Pain can go away after treatment or it can last for weeks, months, or even years. Pain is a major symptom in a lot of medical conditions. When present, it can interfere significantly with quality of life. Pain can be self-limiting or it can respond to simple treatments such as resting, taking painkillers, using hydrotherapy, and physical therapy.

Chronic pain is an emotional condition and a physical sensation that has an effect on thoughts and behavior. Pain can lead to isolation, immobility, and possible drug or alcohol addiction. Pain and depression are similar and have a direct relationship. Pain can cause depression and depression can have an effect on and intensify the pain. The relationship between depression and pain can be found in the brain pathways and is linked with the circuitry of the nervous system. Pain and depression can feed off of each other by altering brain function and behavior. Recent research links depression and pain because both share the same common chemical pathways. Serotonin and norepinephrine play a role in depression and neurotransmitters mediate pain.

Depression is common among injured athletes and they may feel isolated, experience a loss of identity, and may be unsure about their future. Many professional athletes do get injured and go into a depression. Professional skier Picador Street broke her left leg and blew out her right knee in Switzerland in a skiing crash. She went through a depression where she would not talk to family or friends and stayed in her darkened room for weeks. What created a lot of the depression was the fact that it took 20 months for her to recover. In The New York Times, Street mentioned that she felt very isolated due to the combination of the atrophying of her legs, the new scars, and the immobility. She went from being a physical person and an athlete to barely having any strength to get from her room to the kitchen. She felt very secluded and could not do what she normally would do and it made her feel upset and depressed.

Some athletes can remain depressed until the injury has healed. The time period of depression can last for weeks or months and athletes can either attempt or commit suicide because of the depression. Depression can be seen as weakness in an athlete because mental and physical toughness is important to the sport. Injury, pain, and depression can affect self-esteem and quality of life. Seeking a psychologist or sport psychologist can be very helpful in sorting out emotions and neutralizing pain and depression.

When you are injured it is natural to feel depressed over the seemingly unfairness of your condition. You may ask yourself, "Why me?" Dwelling on the situation does not speed up recovery. The goal is to recover and find a way to stay positive from injury to recovery. It is important to stay as strong mentally as you can and ease back into the activity with realistic goals. Take it one step at a time and your body will heal at the rate it is supposed to. It is hard to see the top if you are stuck at the bottom. Overcoming an injury can be like an endurance race in itself. Educate yourself about how the body is repaired and what treatments are necessary for your full recovery.

Self-treatment is very important; however, you should know when to seek professional treatment. Some examples of self-treatment include: hydrotherapy, massage, rest, and possibly over-the-counter anti-inflammatory medication. With a minor injury, pain is usually intermittent and can usually be treated with self-treatment but an injury that is constant and painful can be chronic if not treated properly. You should see a doctor if the pain is severe and constant and you should get a proper diagnosis before starting on a treatment plan. A sports medicine doctor or orthopedist is important if you have a repetitive strain syndrome. A good chiropractor is an important addition to your healing. Chiropractors are both well educated about injuries and the process of how your body heals. A good medical doctor is an essential tool to assist your healing. Your doctor should ask questions about your life as a massage therapist. For example, how many massages do you do in a day, how long have you been doing massage, and what techniques make the pain worse? Also, a good doctor will not only look at the site of injury, he/she will look at the related areas to see if there is some correlation. The doctor will decide on the diagnosis and course of action. This should include a reduced workload or time off completely to heal. Sometimes with your occupation, light duty is not feasible if the injury has become chronic. Complete time off is sometimes necessary to heal completely and correctly. You may be referred to a physical therapist or occupational therapist to regain strength and mobility.

A conservative approach is important with repetitive strain syndrome. Conservative treatment is effective if initiated early enough after the symptoms are felt. Treatments that included massage therapy, stretching, and strengthening can give positive results to patients. Surgery should be considered as your last option and you should definitely get a second opinion if this is the route you decide to take. Be proactive with your recovery.

The best treatment for repetitive strain syndrome is prevention. Nevertheless, injuries can happen, so do not ignore symptoms when they occur. Once an RSI has developed, it is difficult to treat and can last for months and possibly years. Some alternative forms of treatment include: Alexander Technique, Rolfing, Hellerwork, acupuncture, craniosacral therapy, osteopathy, chiropractic techniques, reiki, and nutritional therapies. More often than not a combination of orthodox treatments and alternative therapies are most effective for treating this type of injury. Also, full body relaxation and meditation can help to reduce overall stress and tension in the body and assist in the healing process.

Consider seeing a counselor or go to a support group if you are having problems coping with the pain. Know that fatigue is normal when your body is healing. Give yourself a break and allow nature to take its course and heal your body. Get rest, eat well, and stretch your body. Try not to be a victim and be in charge of your treatment and recovery. Be realistic and keep expectations to a minimum. Play it safe and gently increase your workload until you gain your strength back. If you take a short break now, it may save you from having to take a long break because of a chronic injury later.

Get to know your pain patterns because it helps tremendously with the management of the injury. Also, write a journal on what makes the pain better or worse so you are aware. Be careful not to overdo or overuse the injured body part because this might set you back on your way to recovery. Setbacks are frustrating, but they are very common. Realize that hills and valleys will represent your healing and you have to be patient and ride out the wave. You may be fearful of doing certain activities, especially ones that created the injury. Be gentle with yourself and allow frequent breaks to rest your body. Remain positive even though sometimes it is easier said than done. Try not to become the injury and do not let it control your thoughts and feelings. Try to enjoy the experience; good things always come out of tragedies. Once you are on the other side and healed from your injury, you will have a new outlook on life and a new sense of yourself.

You are at risk for injury when your workload is suddenly increased or the amount of rest time in between your clients is decreased. If you have been off work, increase your workload gently until the body part is back to normal. Schedule clients over time and give yourself more time in-between appointments until your stamina is built back up.

It is smart to think about what you would do financially if you were injured doing your job. Think ahead and contact an insurance agent to get specific details. It depends if you are employed by a company or self-employed. If you are self-employed, you need good health insurance, at least three months worth of income in the bank, and short and long-term disability coverage. If you are employed with a company, it is smart to have good health coverage, pay extra for short and long-term disability coverage, and know your rights for workers compensation. With workers compensation, it depends on the state as to what the laws are. Check with your insurance agent for a broker that can add coverage just for your hands. Know that short and long-term disability covers you if you are injured off the job and workers compensation covers you if you are injured on the job. Know that your case has to be accepted for you to be covered under the workers compensation system.

Accurate medical advice and support is essential to a full and healthy recovery. You may have to deal with pain and other problems such as depression, loneliness, anxiety, workers compensation issues, and possible unemployment. These factors, along with the ongoing pain, can make the recovery process more difficult. Hang in there, educate yourself as much as possible, and seek professional advice when needed. Believe that you will be OK and see yourself healed.

Tips to remember when dealing with the injury process:

- Learn to recognize the body's signs of injury.
- Let healing occur completely.
- Use self-treatment techniques to assist the healing process.
- Know that and depression can occur with pain and seek professional assistance.
- Avoid reinjury.
- Try to prevent an injury from occurring in the first place.

Chapter Ten

The Healing Process

What is physical health? Physical health is the overall condition of your body at a given time, freedom of disease or abnormality, and a condition of well-being. Health occurs when your body functions at the most favorable level. In opposition, disease happens when certain parts of the body become damaged due to injury or illness. Healing is the physical process of the body that repairs and regenerates damage. Healing restores the body to homeostasis and optimal health.

When an injury occurs, recovery is very individual and can take time and patience. Techniques such as massage therapy, relaxation, visualization, positive thinking, rest and sleep can assist the healing process. Receiving massage therapy can be of great benefit to you if you are injured. One of the most important effects of massage is increased circulation. Prolonged muscle contraction can lead to muscle fatigue and massage helps to reduce muscle spasm and contractions. It also assists in breaking down scar tissue in muscles and in the tendons. Massage aids in supplying more oxygen to the area, flushing out waste products, and maintaining flexibility. A pliable muscle can quickly respond to the demands of contraction and relaxation. A positive result of massage is the release of pain-killing endorphins. Massaging the skin helps to release peptides that relax the mind and improve health. You know the benefits of massage and the many different types. You must decide which one is best for your condition.

Massage can definitely help to heal the body. The four stages of healing with massage include: relief, correction, strengthening, and maintenance. During the first few sessions, the goal is to reduce tension and relieve pain. When pain is relieved, the underlying cause can be worked on to correct the problem and free up adhesion and scar tissue. Massage can strengthen the surrounding tissues allowing for more support once the injury has healed. The final stage of healing with massage therapy is maintenance. The final stage is prevention care for the future.

Friction massage is used to work deep into the muscles or around bony prominences. Friction breaks down scar tissue and fibrosis and also increases circulation to soft tissue. Friction increases heat in the tissue and it increases the rate of exchange between the cells and the interstitial fluid. The heat and energy caused from the friction affect the connective tissue by making it more pliable and efficient. This type of massage involves short, deep strokes using solid contact with the underlying tissue. Superficial tissues are massaged against deeper tissues. Friction massage is done using the fingertips, palms, and knuckles. The therapist using friction massage will press down at an oblique angle and rub back and forth in a parallel, transverse, or circular manner. Little or no oil is used with this type of massage.

The different types of friction massage are longitudinal fiber, local cross fiber, and circular friction. Longitudinal friction moves in the same direction as the tissue. It stretches muscles and separates the collagen fibers. Local cross fiber massage is either transverse or crosswise. Cross fiber massage is used on muscle, tendon, and ligament. It helps to increase blood flow, smoothes out scar tissue, and breaks down adhesion. Cross fiber massage is the favored form of massage for rehabilitation. The injury has to be sufficiently healed and scar tissue has to be formed to utilize this technique. The process of scar tissue formation is very important since the support has to be formed before realigning it. After the injury is adequately healed, transverse friction will assist with realignment of fibrous tissue. As a result, the adhesions are broken down and the area will have more strength and pliability. This flexibility of soft tissue will reduce the chance of re-injury.

Transverse friction is especially useful for healing tendons. The intention with this type of massage is to move one layer of tissue over another deeper layer and break up the adhesions. Deep friction is especially good for tendonitis and helps to heal the tendon faster by enhancing the body's natural production of fibroblasts. Thereafter, blood flow is increased and inflammation is eventually reduced. On the other hand, circular friction can be used to warm up and prepare an area for deeper work. Circular friction is quite valuable for releasing painful and spasmed muscles and it also assists in releasing trigger points.

A specific example of applying cross fiber friction to a strained muscle is to let the scar tissue form and then when the area is ready, find the exact site of injury through range of motion and palpation. Apply direct cross fiber friction massage to the exact site of injury for two minutes. Make sure the pressure is within the client's comfort zone and then take two minutes off. Perform cross-fiber friction up to three times, two minutes at a time with two minutes off in between. You can get massage on this area every other day or with two days left in between. Each treatment should be followed by ice massage and gentle range of motion. Fill up a small paper cup two thirds full of water and freeze, then rip off the top of the cup and move the ice in small circles continuously around the area until it melts. Generally, this process of ice massage will take around five minutes. Friction massage should not be used in acute conditions or cases of rheumatoid arthritis, bursitis, or nerve related disorders.

The main goal of healing is to relieve pain, reduce inflammation, and relax connective tissue. It is also important to re-educate your posture and movement. Exercise should not be done until scar tissue is stable and developed. Gentle stretching can be started to realign scar tissue and make the tissue more pliable. Exercise can be added when the injury is healed and inflammation has dissipated.

Repair of the body's tissues will require additional resources to complete the healing process. Adequate amounts of rest, hydration, nutrition, and vitamins are essential during this process. Vitamin C is necessary for fibroblasts to be converted into collagen fibers. Did you know that rosehips have 20 to 40 percent more vitamin C than an orange? When I had my ankle surgeries, I drank rose hip tea and I believe that it helped me repair at a faster rate. In addition to nutrition and vitamins, receiving massage therapy at the appropriate time can help the body's tissues to repair. You should definitely receive massage therapy after the acute phase because it can facilitate healing and restore movement. Massage therapy also increases circulation, delivers nutrients, and eliminates waste products from the area.

Relaxation and visualization can be an important addition to the healing process. The mind and body function as one complete unit. Stress can play a major role in how fast the body heals. The key to controlling stress is to manage it with relaxation. Active relaxation focuses on calming the mind and the body to assist in the healing process. With this technique, you turn your attention inward for awareness and stress relief. Relaxation is the state of mental and physical reprieve when tension, fear, and anxiety are replaced with calm and peace. True relaxation is an acquired skill.

One way to achieve relaxation is to use visualization. You can use your mind to create positive images to heal a part of your body or life. Visualization can include using a favorite scene or a remembered image to help counteract negative thinking. You can use your mind to retreat to a certain place, such as a beautiful beach, tranquil lake, or tropical island. You will relax by lying down or sitting with your eyes closed. Use all of your senses to explore the space you are in. Smell the flowers, feel the temperature, hear the birds sing, and feel a calm breeze against your skin. Once you establish your special place you can relax into it and achieve your goals. A relaxed mind is receptive and open to positive thinking and imaging. Take time to breathe deeply and when you are ready, slowly come out of your visualization session. Use positive affirmations to create an optimistic mindset and use visualization to envision yourself as healthy and strong. See white light flowing to the area that is in need of healing and see yourself using the body part in a normal manner without pain.

Once basic relaxation is achieved, deeper relaxation techniques can be implemented. Hypnotherapy, biofeedback, and meditation are useful for deeper relaxation. I prefer meditation because it frees the mind of excessive thoughts and no goals are set with meditation. The goal is to observe your thoughts and let them float by just like clouds in the sky. The main objective is to achieve inner peace and harmony. Additionally, passive acceptance of yourself is very important to keep in mind and can be a positive by-product to the process of meditation.

Relaxation and visualization are safe for anyone to use. By focusing your attention on what is happening inside the body and mind, you free yourself from outside concerns. Relaxation frees your mind from stress and relaxes the muscles. The parasympathetic nervous system is activated and allows for rest and repair. Visualization promotes right-brained activity and uses the images you provide to override the possible destructive thoughts of the left-brain. If you give your mind a strong and positive image, it will accept it and your goal can be attained.

Always think positive thoughts of healing. Sometimes you have an off day when you are healing. Expect ups and downs, but do not think of yourself as a victim and try to keep your mind in a positive space. Converse with the healing body part and see what it needs. Do not beat yourself up; practice self-acceptance until you are completely healed. Injuries are best treated with respect and constant care. Become aware of how you use your body in all of your daily activities

Sleep is a deep state of rest when tissue regenerates and repairs. It prepares the body for new activity. Most people undervalue rest as an aid for regeneration and healing. Sleeping is a period when emotional, mental, physical, and sensory activity slows or ceases. This time allows the body to redirect its energy into a state of restoration.

You are considered well when the mind, body, and spirit are all balanced. Developing a wellness program is essential to having a healthy massage and bodywork career. A wellness program would include any techniques that will lower stress, repair, and rejuvenate the body. Get to know your responses to stress and the warning signs your body gives you. If there is too much stress on your body as a whole, realize that rest is required. If you do not rest on your own, the body may become depleted and you can develop an illness. Massage is an important part of any wellness program because it restores the balance to all of your systems and gives you the gift of touch.

You know the benefits of massage and touch therapy. Regular massage releases emotional tension, but most important for you as a therapist, getting massage promotes physical health and creates balance in your body. Contracted muscles reduce circulation because they restrict blood vessels. Receiving massage to overused muscles will stimulate circulation, relax muscles, and carry away metabolic waste products. Massage allows the muscles to work in a more efficient and healthy manner.

Allowing yourself time for maintenance massage is very important to the healing process and prevention of injury. It is surprising to me how few therapists allow time for regular massage of their body. Therapists expect self-care from their clients, but often do not take their own advice. Your clients cannot benefit as much if you are not taking care of yourself and are depleted emotionally and physically. Massage may seem like a luxury or you may think that you do not have the time, but you do have a choice. Massage is a necessity for therapists. You should do at least as much for yourself as you do for your clients. Receiving massage keeps you in touch with your own body and provides an evaluation tool for emerging or existent strain patterns. Find your way to a massage table once a week. If this is not feasible, then get a massage at least every other week. You will definitely see and feel the difference. If you are getting maintenance massage, you will feel good suggesting regular massage to your clients. You will ask no more of your clients then you ask for yourself. Be the best therapist you can be and find time to get a massage. Your health is the best assurance you can give to your client. Taking care of yourself is the best guarantee that you will provide your clients with the greatest care possible.

The truth about healing is that it's not just a science; it is a way of living. It should be your way of life and should happen at all times, not just when you are ill. A healthy life requires that your thoughts reflect your needs. By managing your thoughts, you can live a healthy life. If you experience illness, it is time to look inside yourself and evaluate your life. If you are healthy, you should examine your thoughts as a preventive measure. Healing requires you to develop your intuition since it is your guidance system and will help you to read what your physical and energetic bodies are telling you. Healing allows you to live a life full of grace, gentleness, gratefulness, and love.

Look at the physical body as if it were the tip of the iceberg. There is a lot that lies beyond the surface to determine health. Unless you become ill, you may not even be aware what is below the surface. Good health is more than just addressing the physical body and health. It also includes the mind and spirit. The layer below the surface has to do with your behavior, how you act, how you interact with others and how you manage stress. Below this layer is where your beliefs lie. Beliefs are repetitive thoughts that become fixed in your mind and in your behavior. Beliefs are accountable for the habits and comfort zones that form and are hard to change. The mind will support these beliefs because they think they are truth. The next layer below beliefs is the emotional level. This layer contains emotions and attitudes. Herein lays your outlook on life and your inner child. This is also the location of your fears and self-esteem. This layer affects your beliefs and can result in destructive behavior. The layer below emotions is your mental state. If your main thoughts are in agreement with your spirit and the needs of the body, the iceberg will withstand hard times. If the thought patterns are unhealthy and not in alignment, then the foundation will not be strong enough to hold up and remain stable. The main part of the iceberg that is infrequently noticed is the layer of spirit. It is made up of the energy body and soul. This is the largest section that is the foundation of healthy mental, physical, and emotional states. It contains the healing powers that can transform and transcend disease. The spiritual layer provides guidance to restore health and create wholeness. The spiritual layer is where love, faith, and hope reside. These feelings are powerful and can produce change in the energy body to return balance in all other layers.

The healing powers that reside in the spiritual layer are only available if the layer of thoughts accepts its existence and trusts that it can help to heal. All it takes is your willingness to change your thoughts. Believe that you are well and prioritize your life for healing and what is best for you as a whole. Remember that faith, hope, and love are the components needed to live a healthy life.

Tips to help you through the healing process:

- Be patient and take all necessary steps to heal yourself.
- Be proactive.
- Use visualization, positive thinking, and relaxation.
- Receive massage therapy at the appropriate time.
- Be patient and know that healing is a process.
- Have faith and believe that you will heal.

Chapter Eleven

Using Hydrotherapy

Hydrotherapy is defined as the use of water, in any of its forms, for the maintenance of health or the treatment of disease. Hydrotherapy uses the effects of temperature on the body. Hydrotherapy is an ancient technique used by many cultures including the Egyptians, Chinese, Greeks, and Native Americans. This type of therapy is one of the oldest known. Hippocrates used hydrotherapy extensively as a healing modality around 400 BC.

Most therapists focus on hydrotherapy as the external use of hot and cold. Hydrotherapy is a powerful tool, if used properly. The temperature, duration, and extent of each treatment are important to the result. Knowledge of the physiological principles is important for the treatment to be effective.

Water has special healing abilities that are helpful in reducing stress and revitalizing the body. Water is holistic medicine that benefits the whole body and helps the body heal by restoring energy flow. It has distinctive properties that add to its effectiveness as a healing agent. Water has the capability to be a great conductor of heat and can be used internally or externally, has the capacity to alter its states within a limited, yet obtainable temperature range, and it can be used in a solid, liquid, or vapor stage. Water has a hydrostatic effect and the body feels weightless when fully submerged. Hydrotherapy is used to tone up the body, stimulate digestion, increase or decrease circulation, encourages the immune system, and gives relief from pain. The use of hydrotherapy affects the skin and muscles and calms the lungs, heart, stomach, and endocrine system by affecting the nerve reflexes on the spinal cord.

The healing effects that hydrotherapy has on the body are based on the mechanical or thermal effects. This therapy makes use of the body's reaction to hot or cold. The nerves carry impulses felt at the skin deeper into the body to affect the immune system, circulation, and stress hormones. The density of water is similar to that of the human body and when the body is immersed in water, a hydrostatic effect takes place and increases venous and lymph flow. Water is easily accessible, universally obtainable, and is applied quite easily.

The physiological effects of hydrotherapy are thermal, mechanical, or chemical. Thermal effects are created by the application of water at temperatures above or below that of the human body. The greater the variant from body temperature, the greater the effects produced. The mechanical effects are created by the impact of water on the surface of the body, in the case of friction or whirlpools. The chemical effects are noticed when taken internally. The most commonly used method of hydrotherapy that is administered by a therapist is the thermal method.

The goal of hydrotherapy is to normalize the quantity and quality of blood flowing to the tissues. At certain times, an increase in circulation is needed and at other times a decrease in circulation would be required. Hot water can relax a contracted muscle while an ice pack will limit swelling in a particular area. Healing is not caused by the response of the water, but by the reaction of the organism to the application of hot or cold. When applying hydrotherapy, you must have knowledge of the basic physical concepts of the physiological effects produced by the various hydrotherapy techniques.

The circulatory system serves as a transport for blood between the body cells and various organs. This system is also connected to the external environment. The circulatory system supplies oxygen and nutrients to all tissue cells, removes waste products, and is vital to your survival. The basic variations of blood movement through the body are increased or decreased blood flow to an area of the body or through an organ, increased volume of blood in an anemic area, and decreased volume of blood in a congested area of the body.

Hydrotherapy has to do with both the temperature of the water and of the client. Temperature variation and physiology are very important when working with hydrotherapy. Keep in mind that the temperature of the human body is normally 98.6 degrees Fahrenheit, although it can vary throughout the day. The range of temperatures used with hydrotherapy treatments range from very cold to very hot. Think about what you are trying to achieve to get the most out of each treatment.

Various temperatures for hydrotherapy in Fahrenheit:

Very cold	32-55	degrees	Painfully cold
Cold	55-70	degrees	Tolerable, but uncomfortable
Cool	70-80	degrees	Produces goose bumps
Tepid	80-90	degrees	Slightly below skin temperature
Warm	92-100	degrees	Comfortable
Neutral	94-97	degrees	Around skin temperature
Hot	100-104	degrees	Tolerable, but skin turns red
Very hot	104-110	degrees	Can tolerate for short periods

Heat may be transferred from one object to another by conduction, convection, and conversion. Therapies in a massage setting are most often produced by conduction. Conductive heating is the transfer of heat from one point to another without perceptible movement in the conducting medium. Most of the time, direct contact takes place between the source and the tissues. Superficial heat is generally conductive heat and would be utilized in the method of an immersion bath, pack, or compresses.

Applications of hydrotherapy produce reflexive responses that happen because of the nervous system's reaction to the application. Different physiological and reflex effects depend on the temperature used on the body. When using hydrotherapy, physiological effects take place so the body can return to a stable state.

When heat is applied to the body, physiological effects take place to avoid an increase in body temperature. Short applications stimulate the body, whereas, a treatment of longer duration will sedate the body. Thermotherapy is known as the external application of heat for therapeutic purposes. The effects produced by applying heat depend on the mode, temperature, and duration of the application and the condition of the client. Vasodilation and increased blood flow occur when heat is applied to the body. Warm blood from the core will flow to the local tissues. Using heat will sedate, quiet, and soothe the body in most conditions. Applying heat will also relax the muscles, decrease muscle spasms, increase range of motion, and increase oxygen consumption in the body's tissues. Heat is indicated for relief of chronic pain due to a musculoskeletal injury. In the case of an acute injury, heat will increase blood flow and inflammation to the area and should be avoided in treating acute injuries.

Cryotherapy is the use of external applications of cold for therapeutic purposes. The effects of cold are consistent and depressant in nature and depend on the specific application. The local effects of cold are vasoconstriction, which decreases local circulation and tissue metabolism. As the body reacts to the cold application, a state of increased activity is noted as the body returns to normal functioning. If the cold application is of short duration, the response follows quickly. The intensity of cold reflects the intensity of the application. The secondary effects occur when the body responds to the cold, particularly after the body has warmed after the application. Generally speaking, the colder the application, the greater the response. In hydrotherapy, the goal with most cold techniques is the reaction to the cold. Cold applications may be applied with ice, cold water, or the evaporation of water or other liquids from the surface of the body. A short application of cold is stimulating and reduces fatigue.

The phases of a cold application to a particular area start with pain, proceed to burning, then advance to tingling, and end with a numb sensation. Go through the feeling phase, hold in the numb phase for a minute, and then remove the application. Only when you move into the numb phase are you creating a physiological response in hydrotherapy. If the cold application is left until the numb phase, then the contraction of blood vessels is followed by dilation to push out all the waste products. Ice is very important in reducing pain and inflammation. An important effect of applying ice for chronic pain is the reduction of nerve conduction velocity. Ice is the preferred treatment in treating acute injuries and is also a great anesthetic.

Generally, heat increases metabolic rate and tissue pliability. In contrast, cold decreases metabolic rate and tissue pliability. A short duration of ice or heat is 15 to 20 minutes at a time. Ice for 15 minutes, no longer than 20 minutes at a time, and make sure to have a layer between the ice and the skin to avoid frostbite. Ice will help in the retention of fluids and internal hemorrhage of the tissue.

Common methods of application consist of a hot or cold pack, therapeutic baths, and friction treatments. A pack is used for a local hydrotherapy treatment and can be in the form of a gel, compress, clay, or chemical. One of the most valuable hot packs is a hydrocollator pack. These packs are heated in a hydrocollator, which is a small metal tank that uses water heated to 150-160 degrees Fahrenheit. This pack is filled with clay, is good for moist heat, and can retain heat up to 30 minutes. Hydrocollator packs covered with a thick towel are useful to relax hypertonic muscle tissue before you massage an area. Gel packs, homemade ice packs with water and rubbing alcohol, or even a frozen bag of peas can be used efficiently as a cold pack. Cold packs are used with a thin layer on the skin for 15 minutes every hour. Water can be frozen in a paper cup and the corners can be torn off to hold the base and massage an area. With ice massage, move the ice continuously as you massage. This type of hydrotherapy is considered more local instead of systemic in the effects because of the application of short duration.

ICE, ICE, ICE to prevent injury or to lessen injury if it has already occurred. I make it a rule to always ice my arms if I perform more than a few hours of massage in a day. I ice my arms in a two-gallon water thermos, with my arm up to my elbow, in ice water for 15 to 20 minutes as I watch television. I make sure to wait until after the numb phase to remove my arm so the area has relieved the waste products thoroughly. Ice no longer than twenty minutes every hour because prolonged cold can have the reverse effect. You can also do an ice bath with the temperature around 32 degrees Fahrenheit. The treatment time for an ice bath should be from 20 seconds to two minutes because of the intensity of cold.

Applying ice is one of the most important prevention methods I can address. If you are doing more than a couple of hours of massage a day, than you are creating microtrauma and inflammation. Repetitive action creates strain, tension, and inflammation. Therefore, you should ice and stretch immediately after massaging. This technique will prolong your career. Additionally, I add Epsom salt and apple cider vinegar to my bath to relieve aches and pains. If I want to reduce inflammation to an area, I will pound and bruise a leaf of cabbage and wrap the area with plastic wrap and a towel for 15 to 20 minutes.

If injured, ice immediately after the injury to the area of pain. Use the acronym R.I.C.E (Rest, Ice, Compression, and Elevation) to reduce swelling and start the healing process. After the initial phase of injury is over and inflammation is decreased, alternating hot and cold can be helpful. Contrast applications consist of alternating hot and cold to the same area of the body. A vascular flush is created as tissues are pumped and rid of waste products, as a result of vasoconstriction and vasodilation of the blood vessels. The effects of hot and cold contrast are stimulating and increase local circulation. The length of a contrast bath is still under debate. The cold immersion should only be long enough to create vasoconstriction. This occurs in less than a minute. The treatment time is generally three minutes of heat and up to a minute of cold. The treatment consists of doing contrasts of hot and cold, alternating three to five times each. Start with cold and end with cold. A longer contrast can be utilized with a ratio of 10 to 15 minutes of alternating hot and cold. Always end with cold. Reflex effects of contrast therapy have the effects of both hot and cold, but with improved results due to the differences between applications and temperatures.

Heat can relax musculature, warm up tissue, and reduce muscle spasm. Heat helps with chronic conditions to increase circulation to the affected area. Use moist heat on your client to release tight muscles. Use clay packs, water bags, or warm steam towels to reduce tension. The heat will do the warm up work and allow you to penetrate easier under the surface tension. Heat enhances the circulatory process and promotes healing. Avoid heat if there are any signs of inflammation, heat, or redness.

A Paraffin bath is a local application of paraffin wax applied to the skin surface. Paraffin delivers heat effectively to the joints and soft tissue, in addition to, leaving the skin soft and smooth. Paraffin also promotes hyperemia to the tissues. To use paraffin, disinfect your hand and place it in a paraffin bath. Dip the area five to seven times and cover with plastic wrap, then wrap in a towel or paraffin glove. The paraffin can also be applied with a brush, especially if you are working on a large surface area. The treatment time is 20 to 30 minutes, subsequent to the area being wrapped up. Make sure that the temperature of the paraffin does not exceed 130 degrees Fahrenheit. The temperature of the paraffin should be from 122 to 130 degrees. Use a standard paraffin bath and thermometer for temperature regulation. Paraffin is a great treatment applied pre-massage for pain relief and to increase range of motion. The use of paraffin as a self-care treatment is recommended for you as a therapist. Paraffin keeps your skin soft and decreases joint pain. Many people can benefit from using paraffin but there are some contraindications such as hypertension, diabetes, inflamed arthritis, open cuts, dermatitis, and allergies to oils or certain scents.

Steam treatments can be incorporated as an additional treatment, in combination with your massage. Adding steam to your massage can help your client to detoxify their body, warm and hydrate the tissues, and improve the immune system. A steam canopy or cabinet can be purchased from $900 to $2500. A steam cabinet could add to the number of clients you can schedule. You could have a client in the steam cabinet for 20-30 minutes and add an extra $30 to $40 on to your massage session. You could incorporate a steam canopy to the massage and save your hands for 10 minutes a session or you can add 30 minutes of steam for an additional $25. The steam will help your client to relax, release their muscle tissue, and detoxify their body. Make sure your client checks with a health care professional before beginning a steam treatment. Contraindications for steam are individuals with cardiovascular conditions, diseases related to a reduced ability to sweat, defibrillators, and women who are pregnant.

Hydrotherapy has physiological and reflexive effects on the body. Know your client's medical conditions, as hydrotherapy treatment can be powerful in its effects. Hydrotherapy could be contraindicated for clients with circulatory, nervous system, heart, or systemic conditions. Also, clients with skin conditions, decreased sensation, or weakened immune systems should be assessed and cleared by a doctor before hydrotherapy is administered.

The decision to use hot or cold can be confusing, so it is important to understand the physiological responses when using hydrotherapy. The decision to use hot or cold can vary according to the "freshness" of the injury. If the injury is recent, from the time of injury to 72 hours after, then the R.I.C.E principle applies. Ice is the recommended treatment at this time because it can decrease swelling and restrict additional tissue injury. Applying heat during this time period is harmful for the healing process and can worsen the inflammation and increase pain. When the acute period is over, applying heat will help stimulate circulation and encourage healing. Alternating hot and cold can be valuable after the acute stage. Furthermore, heat is beneficial in chronic cases when pain originates from inflexibility of a joint or muscle and ice is advantageous to reduce pain in cases of chronic nerve inflammation. Heat can be used during rehabilitation prior to exercise to increase range of motion and flexibility. Ice that is applied immediately after exercise can reduce pain, decrease inflammation, and assist in healing microdamage that is produced by exercise.

Hydrotherapy is very important for you as a therapist and for you to use on your clients to assist each treatment. Ice and heat both help the injury process along and soften contracted muscle tissue. Furthermore, utilizing hydrotherapy techniques, in addition to strengthening the physical body, oxygenating the tissues, and keeping your energy level high are crucial steps to keeping your body in a healthy state.

Important points to remember when utilizing hydrotherapy:

- Know when it is appropriate to use hot or cold.
- Use the hydrotherapy technique that will make your session most efficient.
- Apply ice when inflammation is present.
- Apply heat to warm up tissue and increase pliability.
- Use contrast baths to rid the area of waste products.
- Make use of hydrotherapy to help prevent injuries.

Chapter Twelve

Posture and Stretching

Posture is defined as the relative position of various parts of the body. Posture is a pattern that is developed by repeating movements over time. It is an important concept to think about when your body is in a sitting or standing position. Correct posture is positioning the body in a way that supports the entire spine, shoulders, hips, and ankles. Proper posture puts less stress on the joints and muscles of the back, hips, and neck. Incorrect posture can cause muscle strain, fatigue, pain, and compression of blood vessels. There are many reasons why you would want to improve poor posture. If you stand leaning forward or slouch when you are seated, you are increasing stress on the joints and the discs. When the body shifts into an incorrect posture, the bones are improperly aligned and the ligaments, joints, and muscles take more stress than is normal.

Good posture consists of the correct alignment of body parts coupled with the right amount of muscle tension in opposition to gravity. Good posture is important because the muscles work more efficiently, thus allowing less energy expenditure and prevention of muscle fatigue. Maintaining good posture and stretching the body go hand in hand. When muscles are more pliable, good posture is easier to maintain. Posture is the position you hold your body in against gravity, while standing upright. Having good posture involves training your body and having constant awareness as to how your body is positioned. The idea of having correct posture is to have a neutral spine. A neutral spine is inherent alignment containing the natural curves of the spine. A healthy spine has three natural curves: a slight forward curve in the cervical area, a slight backward curve in the thoracic spine, and a slight forward curve in the lumbar spine.

To have good posture, it is necessary for your spine, muscles, and joints to be in excellent shape. Good posture means keeping the spines three natural curves in alignment. Strong and flexible muscles are important for good posture. Leg, hip, and abdominal muscles that are weak and inflexible cannot support the natural curves of the spine. The joints of the hips, knees, and ankles should balance the natural curves of the spine when the body is in motion. Upholding good posture helps the body to function more efficiently, have more endurance, and contribute to your general well-being.

Requirements for good posture definitely require muscle balance and flexibility. The postural muscles have to be strong and flexible. Normal motion in the joints is essential or muscle imbalance can occur. Also, awareness is a requirement for good posture. Awareness leads to correction and after time, correct posture will replace any old dysfunctional patterning.

Many factors can contribute to bad posture. Obesity, pregnancy, stress, weak postural muscles, and poor body positioning can pull the body's natural curves out of alignment. Both weak and tight muscles can contribute to poor posture. Also, habits such as incorrect standing and sitting, in addition to, faulty body mechanics when working can create poor posture. A problem that is common to therapists with poor posture is weakness in the lower abdominal muscles. A good way to strengthen the abdominal muscles is to find an exercise that isolates and actively uses all the abdominal muscles at the same time.

Changes in your posture can occur with aging; however, you should continually work at keeping up with your posture. Throughout the day, concentrate on maintaining all three natural curves in your spine and try not to stay in one position for too long. Exercise regularly, keep your weight in check, and protect your back when lifting. Wear comfortable and supportive shoes while you walk with your head erect and your chin level with the ground. Allow your arms to swing naturally and keep the feet pointed straight ahead to concentrate on having correct posture.

Maintaining good posture is a preventive measure. When you have poor posture the muscles, joints, and ligaments are under more strain because the bones are not properly aligned. Incorrect posture can cause muscle strain, fatigue, and pain. Good posture enhances your breathing and circulation. It also contributes to your outward appearance. When you have good posture, you will exude poise, confidence, and pride.

Correct posture is essential to reducing injury and keeps the body open and flexible. A general understanding occurs when you take a look at yourself. Incorrect posture can feel right to you because it is habitual, even though it is not acceptable. Look in the mirror at your spine from the side. Observe your head and neck, and look at how your pelvis is tilted. Notice how your feet contact the ground.

Tight shoulders and a rounded back are very common in the bodywork field. Problems can arise from this type of poor posture. These problems can arise because of the excessive mobility and decreased stability in the shoulder joint. Incorrect posture can be fixed with awareness and allowing the body time to change. Strengthening the core and back muscles as well as, stretching and opening the shoulders are crucial for correcting poor posture.

If you view posture in a holistic way, you will find that posture consists of the way you move, breathe, think, feel, and observe. Holistically, posture has to do with the way you feel in your body. If you are feeling down, your body will sag and when your mood is lifted, your body will be held more upright.

To gain awareness and correct your posture, start by grounding yourself through the feet into the earth. Think yourself tall, feel the feet contacting the floor, and lift the inner arches. Raise the kneecaps to engage the quadriceps and raise the upper body up from the pelvis. Allow the tailbone to fall perpendicular toward the ground. Let the shoulders roll down and back as the spine elongates and your head flows freely up to the sky. Allow the spine to release into its natural curves. A correctly curved spine is stronger, more supple, and can endure gravity better.

If you do the same movements day after day, you develop movement patterns and faulty posture. Stiffness becomes habitual and increases your risk of injury. The human body is very adaptable but the body will compensate and muscle imbalance can occur. Stronger muscles will take over for weak muscles but eventually imbalances can create a repetitive use injury.

Good posture can give you a renewed sense of esteem, prevent injury, and increase oxygen flow to the lungs. Stretching every day, in some way, can contribute to good posture. Relaxation, deep breathing, and stretching can all work together to give you more attention to your own body.

Awareness will help you to discover the areas of stiffness and habitual tension zones so that you can help to erase them and be mindful of where those areas are.

The proper way to sit:

- Keep the feet on the floor
- Position the ankles in front of the knees
- Maintain the knees at hip level
- Relax your shoulders but keep them supported by the back

The proper way to stand:

- Bear your weight on all four corners of your feet
- Keep the feet shoulder width apart
- Maintain a slight bend in the knees
- Hang your arms by the side with the shoulders pulled slightly back
- Keep the abs tucked in
- Make sure your head is in line with the body

Posture and stretching are both important to maintaining the care of your body. Stretching is the deliberate act of lengthening muscles to increase muscle flexibility and joint range of motion. The desire to stretch is natural and instinctive. Stretching relieves physical and mental tension and improves circulation. Stretching, as an exercise, is safe and effective and energizes the whole body. The key is to practice every day. It is very important to practice regularly to be effective.

Before fitness training you must do a warm-up or stretching to increase your flexibility and prevent injuries. Stretching before activity helps you to avoid injury and stretching afterwards will increase flexibility. Holding a stretching position for 20 seconds is efficient for a warm-up and holding a position for 60 seconds encourages the body's flexibility. When you stretch, hold the position for several seconds, relax, and slowly return to the starting position. Do not force your body into a stretch because forcing yourself into a position can damage and stress the joints and muscles.

Stretching is important for many reasons. Stretching helps to keep the muscles healthy and can make you feel better and stronger. Exercises for flexibility help sustain circulation and strength around the joint, especially when performed after a workout or brief cardio warm-up. Stretching allows the body to function more optimally. Muscles tend to shorten as they fatigue during a workout and stretching allows the muscles to be more elongated and reduces the tendency for shortening. Stretching actually makes you stronger when used in combination with exercise. Stretching can increase strength up to 20 percent if done on a regular basis.

It is a good idea to stretch and warm-up all muscle groups. The order in which you stretch is important. When you perform a stretch, you are stretching a particular group of muscles. You should stretch the muscle intended and the supporting muscles. The supporting muscles act as synergists for the main muscle being stretched. It is suggested to stretch the synergist muscles first to allow a better stretch for the primary muscles. For example, to stretch the hamstrings, it would be a good idea to stretch the lower back, gluteal muscles, and the calves first. A good order for stretching would be to stretch the upper and lower back, gluteals, calves, hamstrings, tibialis, quadriceps, arms, and then the chest.

If you stretch properly, you should not be sore the next day. If you are sore, you may be overstretching and very possibly need to stretch less intensely. One of the easiest ways to overstretch is to stretch your muscles "cold" without a warm-up. Stretch within your comfort zone and without pain. Back off if you feel a sharp pain or burning sensation. Stretching should be pleasurable and not painful. Perform each stretch in increments while listening to your body. Stretch to the capabilities of your own body and not of others.

Stretch to warm up the muscles especially on those days when you feel tight, stiff, or when pain is present. Stretch before and after working on each client. A valuable time to implement stretching is when you have done a large number of massages the day before. Develop a daily stretching routine to maintain your body for a long and dynamic career. Stretching on a regular basis increases you range of movement, flexibility, and strength.

Good posture includes:
- Keep the spine in a neutral position by maintaining the three natural curves.
- Sustain strength and flexibility in the muscles.
- Constantly have awareness so you can correct inefficient movement patterns.
- Stretch the chest muscles and strengthening the back and core muscles.
- Continually have awareness of how you move and how you hold your body.
- Uphold balance in all of your muscles.
- Maintain a general understanding of how you feel in the moment.

Points to note when stretching:
- Start with basic stretching.
- Stretch slowly and stretch less to begin with.
- Pay attention to your body while you stretch and keep the spine straight.
- Wear loose clothing, work on a mat or non-slip surface, and stretch a half an hour before and after eating.
- Pay attention to the area you are stretching and tune in.
- Feel your limbs extending as the muscles elongate away from the spine and let the joints move freely.
- Stretch the spine up and extend the head toward the sky, as you feel a lifting sensation in the whole spine.
- Increase each stretch only after you feel the muscle release or relax.
- If you feel pain, then back off.
- Breathe smoothly and evenly as you stretch.
- Come out of the stretch slowly and cautiously.
- Repeat each stretch two to three times.

Chapter Thirteen

Strength Training

Strength training is an important part of a balanced exercise routine and includes flexibility exercises and aerobic activity. Regular aerobic exercise makes the muscles use oxygen more efficiently while strengthening the heart and the lungs. When you do strength training, your muscles are used against resistance. Strength training helps to tone, strengthen, and increase muscle mass.

Doing bodywork requires muscular fitness. Maintaining good physical condition of your body is a part of your job. Muscle strength and endurance are essential components for a healthy career in bodywork. Increasing baseline strength enhances the quality of your work performance and lowers your risk of injury. Resistance training helps to improve both muscle strength and endurance. Strength training involves an overload in the amount of resistance, whereas, endurance calls for an overload in the number of repetitions. When developing your strength, perform each exercise to fatigue/failure with resistance for no less than six to eight repetitions in one to three sets. Precise and specific training improves bodywork performance. If you are performing mostly sports massage, strength or power exercises should include more resistance and bursts of speed with slow eccentric contraction. On the other hand, if you carry out more Swedish and deep tissue strokes for eight hours a day, you want to build stamina by using less weight and more repetitions. A fit therapist should have the capability to use muscles repetitively, over a long period of time, without excessive fatigue.

The type of resistance you use to build and tone the muscles is individual, depending on your goals. You can chose to use your body's own resistance, exercise tubing, free weights, machines and cables, or elastic bands. Relying solely on massage and bodywork to build your strength can be detrimental because certain muscle groups can be overloaded and can create muscle imbalance, which can lead to injury.

Strengthening the upper body involves exercises for the back, chest, shoulders, abdominals, forearms, triceps and biceps. Weight training the upper body will improve your posture and body image. It is suggested that you open and stretch both the pectoralis muscles and maintain the strength of your entire back. Most weight training for bodyworkers should include low weight and high repetitions for muscular endurance.

Proper warm up of the muscles is essential to any exercise program. The purpose of an active warm up is to increase blood flow to the muscles and to increase body temperature. This will make the tissues supple and improve their pliability and range of motion. For a warm up to be effective, carry out movements that slightly increase your heart rate, breathing, and create a light sweat. A proper warm up also primes the nerve to muscle pathway to prepare the tissues for exercise. A general cardiovascular warm up, such as a five-minute walk or jog or a sport specific activity, can serve as an appropriate warm up.

Proper posture and body alignment are crucial when performing these exercises. You should carry out all exercises in a slow and controlled manner. Breathe evenly while performing the exercises and exhale during the most difficult phase of the repetition, making sure not to hold the breath. The exercises listed here are for the arms, shoulders, back, forearms, abdominals, and legs. Always consult your doctor before beginning any physical fitness program. The doctor should evaluate and clear you of any medical conditions. The assistance of an exercise physiologist or a certified personal trainer is also recommended for the beginning of an exercise program. Either professional can assist you in rehabilitating any injuries, meet your fitness demands, and help you with specific problems. After an injury, strengthening should not be done until inflammation has subsided and nerve compression has dissipated.

Dumbbell Shoulder Press
The dumbbell shoulder press strengthens the shoulders, triceps, and upper back. It is also called the overhead press and can be done seated or while standing. This exercise helps to create equal strength in both arms.
1) While seated, keep your back upright with the feet flat on the floor.
2) Hold the dumbbells in each hand at shoulder height with the elbows facing down and the palms facing forward
3) Exhale as you slowly press your arms over your head until the dumbbells almost come together. Be sure not to lock your elbows.
4) Lower the dumbbells back to the original position by your shoulders.
5) Repeat one-three sets of 10-15 repetitions.
Be cautious if you have any elbow, low back, neck, or shoulder injuries. If this exercise or any other exercises cause you excessive pain in the shoulders or numbness and tingling in the arms and fingers, stop immediately. (13.1)

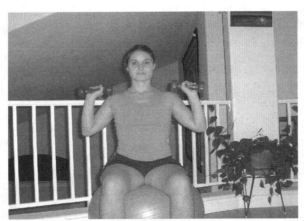
13.1 Dumbbell Shoulder Press

Lateral Raise
The lateral raise strengthens the upper back and shoulder muscles. This exercise helps to build strength while defining the shoulders. The lateral raise is a great exercise for targeting the medial deltoids.
1) Stand with the feet shoulder width apart and your arms by your side.

2) Lift the dumbbells by keeping the palms facing down, with the elbows slightly bent, and raise your arms to shoulder height. Think of leading the movement with the elbows instead of the hands or the wrists.

3) Lower the arms back to starting position and repeat one-three sets of 10-15 reps.

Use proper form with this exercise by keeping the body in alignment with the back straight and the abdominals contracted. The key to this exercise is to keep the elbows slightly bent toward the back of the room instead of the floor. If this exercise is difficult, try this exercise with the elbows bent at 90 degrees to take some strain off the shoulders. Avoid this exercise if you have shoulder, neck, or low back injuries. (13.2)

Front Raise

The front raise works the anterior deltoids and the front of shoulders. This exercise targets the anterior deltoids and other areas of the front of the shoulder. The front raise will assist you with lifting and make it more effortless.

1) Hold light to medium weights with the arms by your side and the palms facing your thighs.
2) Raise your arms out in front of you until the arms are parallel to the floor.
3) Exhale and then lower back to the original position.
4) Repeat one-three sets of 12-16 repetitions with 20-30 seconds of rest in between each set.

Make sure you keep the back straight and concentrate on using only the shoulders to lift. If you want to concentrate on strengthening one shoulder at a time, alternate between the left and right arm to lift each dumbbell. Be cautious with shoulder raises if you have any neck or shoulder injuries. (13.3)

Reverse Fly

The reverse fly or bent over lateral raise works the upper back and tricep muscles to target important muscles for proper posture. You can use the pec fly machine to perform the reverse fly or lean over while seated on a bench or ball. This exercise is important because it allows the muscles of the shoulders to strengthen evenly and helps you to keep the chest open.

1) Hold light to medium dumbbells in each hand and lean over while the arms are hanging down, with the weights under the knees.
2) Keep the back straight and the abdominals contracted as you extend the arms to the side and squeeze the shoulder blades together.
3) Keep the elbows slightly bent, palms facing down, and only lift to shoulder height.
4) Lower your arms back to the starting position and repeat one to three sets for 12-15 reps with a 20-30 second rest in between.

Perform this exercise in a slow and controlled manner with the spine neutral and the abdominals contracted. Keep the movement small and the weights light for this exercise. Avoid this exercise if you have shoulder or neck injuries. (13.4)

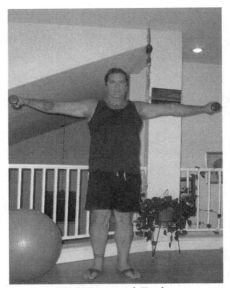
13.2 Lateral Raise

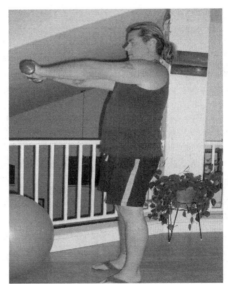
13.3 Front Raise

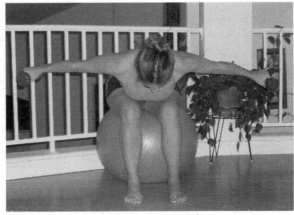
13.4 Reverse Fly

<u>External and Internal Shoulder Rotation</u>

The rotator muscles rotate and stabilize the shoulder joint in the socket. Maintaining strength and endurance in the rotator cuff muscles is very important for bodyworkers because the static postures that are held need to be done with proper stabilization from the muscles. The external rotators are used for stabilizing the shoulder in the socket and to create the action of external rotation. This exercise works the external rotator cuff muscles.

1) Lie on your left side and bend your right elbow to a 90 degree angle next to your side, with your forearm resting on your stomach.
2) Hold a light dumbbell in the right hand with the palm facing down.
3) As you keep the upper arm in a fixed position, raise the right hand in an external motion to the point that feels comfortable.
4) Lower your right hand back to your abdomen.
5) After carrying out a set of 10 to 12 repetitions with the right hand, switch sides and repeat with the left hand. (13.5)

Dumbbell internal rotation is an important exercise for bodyworkers as well. The internal rotator muscles stabilize the shoulder and perform the action of internal rotation.

1) Lie on your right side with your left elbow rested at the side of your body.
2) Hold a dumbbell in your right hand with the right elbow bent at a 90 degree angle and rested on the floor.
3) Keep the upper right arm fixed while you raise the right hand toward your body.
4) Slowly lower the weight back to the original position.

After carrying out a set with the right hand, switch sides and repeat with the left hand. As you lift the arm up, imagine the shoulder moving as a hinge. Keep the body stationary as your arm is in motion and move your arm only as far internally or externally as is comfortable. Light dumbbells or exercise tubing is recommended for this exercise. Rest your head on a rolled towel to prevent straining the neck. Use caution if you have any rotator cuff injuries. (13.6)

<u>Lat Pull down</u>

The lat pull down strengthens the latissimus dorsi, rhomboids, and the rear deltoids. This exercise is essential for a strong back and adds the v-shape to the back.

1) Sit or stand with the back upright and the abdominals engaged.
2) Hold a resistance band or tubing in both hands, above the head, and a little wider than shoulder width.
3) Move the left arm above the shoulder and pull the right elbow down toward the ribcage to contract the lat muscles.
4) Switch to the opposite side and repeat for one to three sets of 10-15 repetitions.

If you are using a machine, keep your back straight and your abdominals tight to protect the back while performing this exercise. Another way to work the latissimus dorsi is to use a yoga strap to perform this exercise. Be careful with this exercise if you have any shoulder, elbow, low back, or neck injuries. (13.7)

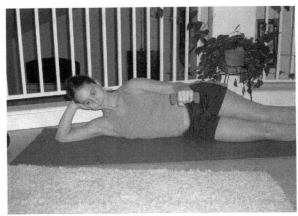

13.5 External Rotation

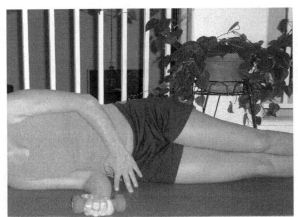

13.6 Internal Rotation

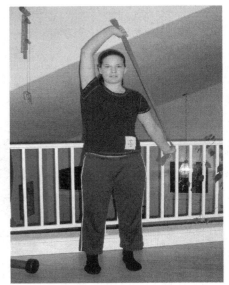

13.7 Lat Pulldown

One Arm Dumbbell Row

The one arm dumbbell row works the latissimus dorsi, back, rear shoulder muscles, and the biceps. This exercise can help correct imbalances in the back muscles. It is important to concentrate on this exercise as a back exercise while you lift the weight.

1) Bend at the waist with the torso parallel to the floor.
2) Keep the knees bent as you hold the weights down by your legs.
3) Lift the weight until the elbow is level with your torso as you keep the shoulder relaxed.
4) Lower your arm down and repeat for one to three sets of 10-15 repetitions and then switch to the other side.

As you perform this exercise, keep the abdominals tight and the spine straight. You should lift only the amount of weight that is comfortable to pull the elbow back and squeeze the shoulder blade to the spine. Another similar exercise you can do is a seated cable row. It is also good for strengthening and creating stabilization for the back. The rowing machine also creates the same action and is a great way to build some cardiovascular endurance. Be careful if you have shoulder, neck, elbow, or low back conditions. (13.8)

Tricep Extension

The tricep extension builds and tones the triceps. This exercise uses both hands to perform the movement and can be done while seated or standing.

1) Sit on a bench or a ball and hold a dumbbell with both hands.
2) Move the weight over the head with the arms next to the ears.
3) Lower the dumbbell behind the head until the elbows are bent to 90 degrees.
4) Straighten the arms while you squeeze the tricep muscles being careful not to lock the elbow joint.
5) Repeat for one to three sets of 10-15 repetitions.

To perform this exercise, do not lock your elbows and keep the spine in a straight line. Position the wrists close together to keep the elbows from moving out to the sides. Keep your neck straight while you look straight ahead. Use caution if you have neck, shoulder, or elbow injuries. (13.9)

Hammer Curl

The hammer curl strengthens the biceps, forearms and the elbow joint. This exercise is comparable to a dumbbell curl, except the hammer curl works a different part of the biceps. It focuses on the forearms and the palms are facing each other instead of facing up.

1) Sit or stand with the feet hip width apart and keep the back straight.
2) Begin with the arms at your side, elbows slightly bent, and the palms facing each other with the thumbs up.
3) Bend your elbows as you move the dumbbells toward the shoulders with the palms facing each other.
4) Slowly lower the arms back to your side.
5) Repeat one to three sets of 10-15 repetitions.

To perform this exercise, keep your back in neutral position, head facing forward, and your elbows close to your body. If you want to focus on one arm at a time, you can alternate arms. Be cautious if you have any elbow or wrist problems. (13.10)

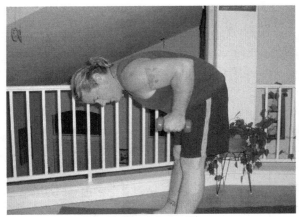

13.8 One Arm Row

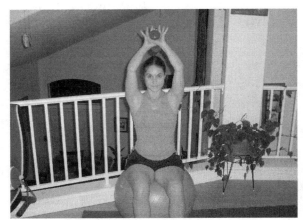

13.9 Tricep Extension

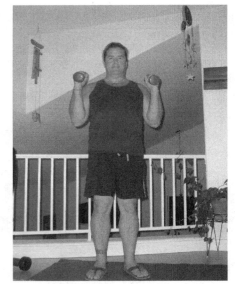

13.10 Hammer Curl

Wrist Curl

The wrist curl is great for strengthening the wrists and forearms. This exercise is important for bodyworkers because it helps to assist with muscle balance in the forearms. Maintaining wrist strength helps you to grasp and grip and is important for preventing injury.

1) Sit on a bench with a light dumbbell in one hand.
2) Bend forward slightly as you rest your forearm on your thigh.
3) As your palm faces up, flex the wrist toward the forearm and lower to the starting position.
4) Switch to a reverse wrist curl by placing the forearm on the thigh with the palm facing down.
5) Extend the wrist toward the forearm and then straighten your wrist back to the neutral position.

To perform this exercise, place the forearm on your leg, keep the abdomen contracted, and the back straight. Use lighter weights and keep the movement slow. Do not perform if you have wrist or hand injuries. (13.11) (13.12)

It is very important for a bodyworker to have a strong core. Your core contains the abdominals and the low back muscles and is at the center of the body. The core is the foundation for all movement, especially the power movements. Core exercises are valuable for improving your posture and building strength so that you will be less prone to injury. A strong core also helps you to stabilize the spine and creates a strong center from which your body can move around. One of the most important paybacks of strengthening the abdominal muscles is that these muscles assist in supporting the low back. If you have existing low back, neck or abdominal injuries, avoid abdominal strengthening exercises until you can check with a professional that can assist you.

Select three-five abdominal exercises to perform two-three times a week. Begin with two sets of 10-15 repetitions for each exercise and work up to three sets of 30 repetitions. Rest a day in between each abdominal workout.

Basic Crunch

Start lying on the floor with your knees bent and the feet flat for the basic crunch. Place your hands behind your head and feel your low back resting on the floor. Slowly allow your abdominal muscles to lift the head and shoulders off the floor. Perform two sets of 30 repetitions. Avoid straining the neck and always use proper form. (13.13)

Bicycle Maneuver

Lie on your back with your knees bent and feet flat to perform the bicycle maneuver. Put your hands behind your head for support and press your lower back into the floor. Bend your knees to a forty-five degree angle and pedal with the motion of riding a bicycle. Bring your right elbow to the left knee and left elbow to your right knee. Continue breathing as you move smoothly and evenly. Perform two sets of 20 repetitions. Be careful with this exercise if you have low back or knee problems. (13.14)

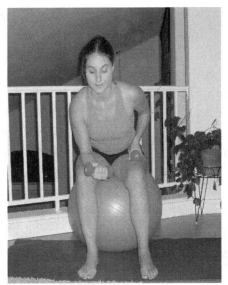

13.11 Wrist Flexion

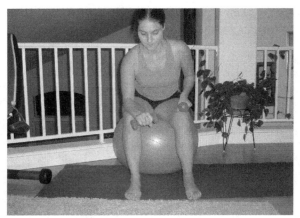

13.12 Wrist Extension

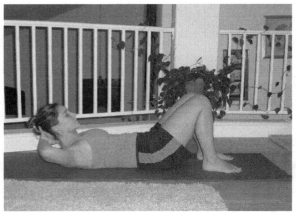

13.13 Basic Crunch

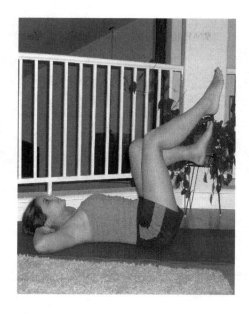

13.14 Bicycle

Crossover Crunch

The crossover crunch is a good exercise for toning and strengthening the sides and the front abdominal muscles. This exercise targets the rectus abdominis, external obliques, and internal obliques. Start on your back with the feet flat and keep your low back on the floor. Lift your head and shoulders off the mat and reach your elbow toward the opposite knee. Slowly lower back to the starting position and alternate with the other elbow and opposite knee. Be sure to keep your neck straight and prohibit your neck from being pulled forward by the hands. (13.15)

Reverse Crunch

The reverse crunch is especially good for working the lower abdominal attachments and the obliques. To begin, lie on your back and place your legs perpendicular to the floor with the feet in the air. Place your arms on the floor next to you. Keep the low back and upper body on the floor as you perform this exercise. Concentrate on raising the buttocks one to two inches off the floor while lifting from the lower abdominals. Hold this position for a few seconds and squeeze your abdominal muscles. Lower slowly back to the starting position. (13.16)

Forearm Plank

The plank works all the abdominal muscles, the shoulders, and the back. It is a core stability exercise and assists with isometric contraction. To start, lie face down on the floor with the elbows shoulder width apart, palms together, and fingers interlaced. Push off the floor with your forearms and lift the hips up. Hold the position for 15 seconds. Lower your hips and rest for 10 seconds before you repeat. You can try a more challenging version by lifting one foot off the floor after you are able to achieve holding the exercise for two minutes. Do not perform this exercise if you have neck, shoulder, or low back problems. (13.17)

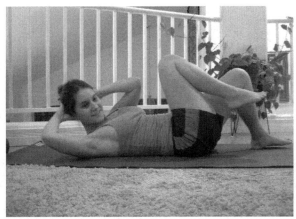

13.15 Crossover Crunch

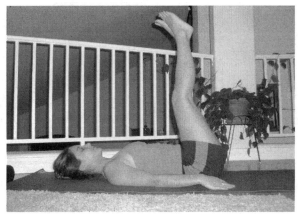

13.16 Reverse Crunch

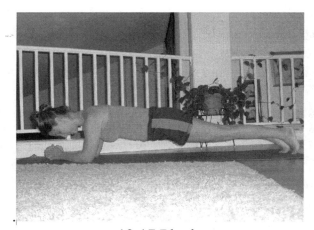

13.17 Plank

Side Plank

Side plank is excellent for targeting the abdominals, the shoulders, and the back. This exercise helps to tone and firm the side abdominals and waistline. Position your body on the side with the legs together and straight. Place your elbows underneath the shoulders and the hands flat. Tighten your abdominals as you lift yourself off the ground with the support of your arm. Lift your body to form a straight line. Hold the position for 10 seconds and lower back to the starting position. Be very cautious of this exercise if you have any shoulder or rotator cuff injuries. (13.18)

Low Back Extension

The low back extension exercise is great for strengthening the muscles of the low back, gluteals, and deep abdominals. This exercise will give you the strength and support needed to protect the low back. A stability ball is a great tool to use for this exercise. To perform low back extension, lie on a stability ball in the face down position. Keep the ball steady as you lift the upper body towards the ceiling to extend the back. Make sure the back is straight and the movement is slow and steady when doing this back extension exercise. Avoid this exercise if you have any acute low back injuries. (13.19)

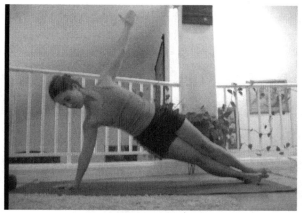

13.18 Side Plank

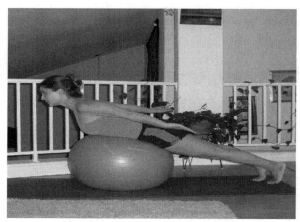

13.19 Low Back Extension

Balance is fundamental when it comes to body mechanics. A sense of balance is the stability produced by even distribution and has to do with weight, force, and influence. Balance helps you to transfer your weight properly. Improving and maintaining balance is crucial for performing bodywork correctly.

During my rehabilitation I discovered the wobble board. The wobble board or core board is an unstable platform that I used to build proprioception and ankle strength. This board can also be used from five to ten minutes a day to increase core strength, stability, and balance. Balance is necessary to deliver a technique with correct weight transference. Bodyworkers with good balance will produce smooth and steady pressure. To start building balance and core strength, find a wobble board that has a non-slip surface and that fits your size and needs. Begin this exercise by holding onto a wall or doorway and then progress with your own body's balance alone. Bring your navel toward your spine as you keep your balance steady and let your body rock in all planes of movement. This helps to build core strength and increases balance and posture. By improving body awareness and proprioception, you will become more efficient and use less energy when working.

A Swiss or stability ball can be used for strength training and stretching. These types of balls are not stable and make the low back and abdominals balance. The size of the exercise ball depends on your height. When you sit on the ball, your hips should be level or a little higher than the knees. You can perform exercises on the stability ball and use the ball instead of a bench for weight training. Many exercises can be performed on a stability ball. The wall squat can be used to strengthen the lower body. The bent over lateral raise, seated dumbbell curl, and external rotation can all be performed on the ball to strengthen the upper body. Also, the basic abdominal crunch, side crunch, and reverse crunch can be worked on the ball to strengthen the core. The back extension exercise can be done on the ball to strengthen the low back and balance out the core strengthening exercises.

Strong leg muscles are essential for a bodyworker's career. The legs are your source of power and have to be strong to maintain the strength and endurance needed for your job. Building strength in the lower body can make standing and applying pressure much easier. A strong lower body can help your balance and lifting will become much more effortless.

The Lunge
Lunges work the quadriceps, hamstrings, buttocks, hip flexors, and gastrocnemious. This exercise improves the balance and strength needed for standing and leaning. You will perform this exercise with weights in your hands or you can just place your hands on your hips. Stand with your feet hip width apart and keep your spine straight. Take a large step forward with right leg and bend both knees to a 90 degree angle. The right knee should not go passed the ankle. Slowly lift your body back to the starting position, pushing through the heel of right foot. When you have completed the set with the right leg, repeat with the left leg. Perform one to three sets of 8-15 reps depending on your fitness level. Do not perform this exercise if you have any knee conditions. (13.20)

Squat
The squat strengthens the gluteals, hips, and thighs. This exercise improves conditioning of the legs because it is a multi-joint exercise. The squat is great for beginners and does not require any equipment. It is a great exercise to use for increased functioning because it copies the movements you do on a daily basis. Place your feet hip width apart and contract your abs as you slowly squat as if you were going to sit in a chair. Keep the knees behind and in line with the toes as you perform the squatting action. Contract the gluteals and abdominals as you lift up out of the position and return

back to standing. If you are unsteady or feel you need extra support, then place a chair behind you. Perform this exercise for one to three sets of 10-15 reps and when you want to make the exercise harder, then squat and hold the position for 30 seconds to a minute. Avoid this exercise if you have knee problems. (13.21)

Kneeling Kickback

The kneeling kickback is a good exercise for toning the hamstrings and gluteal muscles. Rest on all fours on the floor with the abdominals slightly contracted. Place your elbows under the shoulders with your palms facing down. Lift your right leg up with the thigh parallel to the floor and bend your right knee to 90 degrees. Lift the leg up as you contract the gluteals, pause, and return to the starting position with the knee on the floor. Perform this exercise for one to three sets of 10-15 reps and when you have completed the set on the first side, repeat the lift with the left leg. You can add ankle weights or a dumbbell for more resistance. Perform this exercise in a slow and controlled manner and use caution with this exercise if you have knee, shoulder, or low back conditions. (13.22)

Leg Extension

Leg extension strengthens the quadriceps and helps to strengthen the hip joint. It is best to perform this exercise by moving slowly through the full range of motion. Sit against the wall with your legs straight out in front of you. Your hands should remain flat on the floor next to your hips. Keep your legs straight and raise your right leg up and then move it back down to the starting position. Perform this exercise for one to three sets of 10-15 reps. Repeat with the other leg after the set is completed. Keep your back against the wall and avoid this exercise if you have hip, low back, or quadriceps injuries. (13.23)

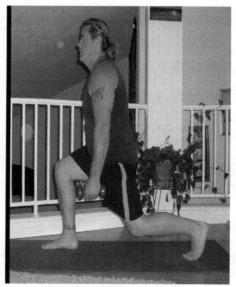

13.20 Lunge

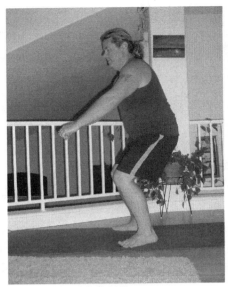

13.21 Squat

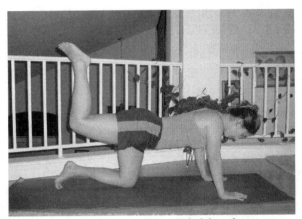

13.22 Kneeling Kickback

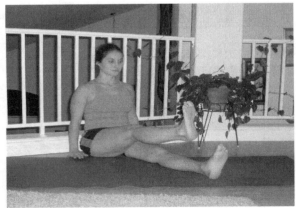

13.23 Leg Extension

In addition to strength training, cardiovascular exercise is an important part of your exercise routine. Cardiovascular exercise helps heart health, circulation, and helps to control weight. Perform cardiovascular exercise three to four times a week for twenty to thirty minutes at a time. Cardiovascular exercise complements weight training by giving the muscles fresh blood and energy. Some common cardiovascular machines are the treadmill, the stationary bike, the elliptical machine, the rowing machine, and the stair climber.

Cross training is a routine that focuses on several different forms of exercise. Cross training conditions different muscle groups and reduces boredom in your workout routine. It varies the stress put on your muscles, tendons, and ligaments. Varying your activities allows the muscles to be used in different ways. It is beneficial to cross train so you can uphold a high level of overall fitness. Cross training will reduce your risk of injury and allow other muscles to rest and recover. Also, this method of training can improve skill, agility, and balance. Different cardiovascular exercises are running, swimming, biking, cycling, rowing, rope jumping, and stair climbing. Strength training routines could vary with calisthenics, machines, free weights, exercise tubing, and stretch bands. In addition, you could include stretching and yoga for flexibility, circuit training, and plyometrics for diversity.

Swimming is excellent for cross training and for injury rehabilitation. Water adds magic to a workout because of the support and resistance it gives to the body and its movement. Water acts like a cushion for weight bearing joints. Water is denser than air and your muscles have to work harder than if you were moving your body through air on land. If you have a sore knee or an elbow that hurts, it is still ok to do gentle water exercises. You can exercise in the shallow end to do basic exercises or work in the deep end for balance, abdominal strengthening, walking, or running. Water is very helpful to help heal certain injuries. After the inflammatory response is over, gentle range of motion exercises can be started in the water. The area around the injury has been de-conditioned after an injury and water is a valuable medium to condition the tissues and rehabilitate. Ask your physical therapist for specific details concerning your injury. During the first phase of rehabilitation, you will concentrate on total body fitness while protecting and possibly immobilizing the injured area. Once you can accept movement of the injured area, you can do more specific rehabilitation exercises. If you cannot tolerate movement of the affected joint, exercise the adjacent joint. If you have pain with a certain exercise either modify it or if it hurts too much, disregard it for the time being. Always increase your workload gently and exercise with the proper biomechanics. Include a warm up and cool down with your therapy. While water therapy is great for the lower body, it is also good for the upper body. Upper body water exercises include movements for the rotator cuff, wrists, elbow, and shoulder.

A proper warm up and cool down are essential to a healthy career and for your workout routine. A proper warm up can increase blood flow and oxygen to the muscles and the range of motion around the joints is increased. The best time to stretch a muscle is after the blood flow has increased in the muscle. Stretching a cold muscle can increase your chances of injury. It is better to engage in gradual aerobic exercise to make the muscles warm and pliable. Five to ten minutes of jogging or biking would help to warm up the muscles. A warm up is very individual and you should try to warm up your body in various ways and find what works best for you.

A cool down is defined as a full body exercise that permits the body to shift from an exercise state to a non-exercise state. Cooling down from running could include jogging or walking. It depends on the intensity of the activity as to what type of cool down you would do. A low intensity exercise could just include stretching. Cooling down helps to decrease muscle tissue temperature and waste products. Five to ten minutes is appropriate for a cool-down. Static stretching is useful for a cool down because it facilitates muscle relaxation and increases range of motion in the joints.

Stretching should be included in every exercise routine to maintain flexibility. Stretching can also improve posture and reduce muscle soreness created from exercise. It is a great idea to make use of stretching before and after exercise and at least three times a week. As you stretch the muscle, relax into the stretch going to first point of resistance. Hold each stretch for ten to thirty seconds and keep the movements slow and smooth. Execute at least one stretch for every major muscle group and breathe as you stretch. You should not feel pain when you stretch and if you do, back out until you feel a good stretch with no pain or discomfort. You can stretch in a doorway to open the chest. Also, gently pull the neck toward the chest to stretch the back of the neck and shoulders. Stretch the forearms by bringing the wrist into flexion and extension. Bring the leg behind you with the knee bent to stretch the quads and bend over at the hips to stretch the hamstrings. Release the hip flexors with a low lunge and relax the calves by pressing your hands against a wall, with one leg back at a time.

You can optimize your workouts and get the most out of every workout with a few easy concepts. For resistance training, focus on every repetition you do and focus your mind on each muscle group, as you feel all the muscle fibers activate with each concentric (lifting of the weight) phase of the repetition. Visualize receiving all the benefits from your workout as you push and pull and with each repetition. See each movement giving your body strength, definition, and power. If you see and feel the phases of strength training, you can trick your body into adapting and working harder. One more tool to make your workouts more productive is to visualize your whole workout from beginning to end; every rep, every set, and every exercise as if you were doing it right then. Now, begin your workout and notice that the adaptation will happen with much less effort.

Use the ten percent rule to increase training and reduce the risk of injury. Increasing the intensity or activity too quickly can increase the risk of injury. To avoid this, increase your exercise by no more than ten percent a week. The ten percent rule includes intensity, distance, timing of exercise, and weight lifted. This rule is a great way to track training and consistency. Listening to your body is the best tool to use. Ignoring aches and pains may put you at risk for serious injury. If your body is giving you warning signs, slow down, modify the exercise, and rest to respect what your body needs. Use this rule not only for exercise, but also as a concept for doing bodywork.

Points to consider when weight training and exercising:

- Always start your exercise with a proper warm up.
- Include resistance training and cardiovascular exercise to maintain strength and endurance.
- Always use proper form when exercising.
- Cross train for efficiency.
- Do a cool down at the end of your workout.
- Use ten percent rule to increase your training.

Chapter Fourteen

Utilizing Your Breath

Everything is connected in the human body. The mind and physical body are linked and can be influenced by each other. Posture and breathing are definitely related and need to be acknowledged when either becomes faulty. People who have poor posture do not understand that incorrect breathing could be connected and individuals that have breathing problems do not look at correcting their posture.

Breath is fundamental to life. The breath is such an essential part of life that movement in conjunction with breathing can be overlooked. The components of the breath keep us alive and consist of an inhale and exhale and an expansion and contraction. Similar to other movements, breathing can be done with grace and efficiency or it can be performed incorrectly and it can be painful. How effectively you inhale and exhale are correlated to how you think, feel, and function physically. How you breathe on a daily basis is both voluntary and involuntary. Most people rarely pay attention to their breath unless a problem occurs. Paying attention to the breath is very useful. It reminds you to be present and more conscious in your body.

Correct breathing is not just about receiving and expelling air out of the lungs. The fundamental movements of breathing are expansion and contraction of the lungs. The inhalation is an expanding movement that draws air inward and the exhalation is a constricting movement that forces air out. Most people breathe in a shallow manner, especially people that are stressed and nervous. Shallow breathing increases the level of carbon dioxide in the bloodstream and can reduce oxygen to the brain and all cells of the body. The average person only uses a portion of their lung capacity because they are not using their diaphragm to breathe.

To understand this, you need to understand basic anatomy of the lungs. The basic purpose of the lungs is to bring oxygen to the blood and remove carbon dioxide from the bloodstream. Your physical and mental health both depend on how much oxygen is delivered throughout the body. The left lung is divided into two parts and the right lung is divided into three. The diaphragm is a muscle that separates the chest and the abdominal cavity. The chest contains the lungs and is protected with the rib cage. Most sedentary people use only the top portion or superior lobe of the lungs. Individuals that breathe in a shallow manner breathe more often and the chest wall does not expand very much. This type of shallow breathing is unproductive because it falls short of exposing the major volume of air to the lungs. With more fit individuals, middle breathing accesses more lung capacity. Even at this point, half of the total lung capacity is not used. Only deep breathing uses the full capacity of the lungs. Deep breathing completely fills and empties the lungs with each inhalation and exhalation. The intercostals muscles move the ribs upward and outward to expand the chest wall as the diaphragm contracts and pulls downward. Deep breathing accesses the lower lobe of the right lung and stale air is expelled out.

The ideal rate for proper breathing is around twelve breaths per minute. When you breathe deeper and more consciously, you have the benefit of delivering more oxygen to your bloodstream and you get rid of large volumes of stale gases. You will also feel more relaxed, as a result. Performing breathing exercises can increase the amount and percent of air you take in. Deep breathing will oxygenate, give energy to the body, and keep your mind focused. Breathing deeply can increase your overall energy.

Posture can have a great effect on your breathing. Slumping the shoulders can decrease the volume of the lungs and can cause shallow breathing. Correcting posture can have amazing results on your breath quality. Proper technique is very important to breathing correctly. Stop, look in the mirror, and take a deep breath. Now exhale. What did you notice? Did your chest and shoulders expand? Did your belly expand? If you were breathing correctly, you would notice the belly expand. Also, the chest would enlarge slightly and the shoulders would remain relatively stable on the inhale. On the exhale, you would examine the chest contracting and the belly moving in toward the spine.

Proper breathing begins with using the diaphragm. The diaphragm moves downward, on the inhale, letting the lungs expand. The abdominal muscles then push the diaphragm up against the lungs to exhale and push all the air out. If the deep abdominal muscles are not well toned, the initiation of the diaphragm on rib cage expansion does not occur as correctly and the rib cage must be expanded by the scalenes and accessory breathing muscles of the upper chest. This type of improper breathing can lead to chronic muscle tension in those areas and affect your posture. Deep breathing uses the diaphragm and rib cage more and the upper chest less. As a result, total lung capacity is considerably expanded and breathing actually becomes easier. Consequently, the body releases endorphins and creates a tranquilizing and relaxing effect on your body.

To start with a deep breathing exercise, visualize your lungs as a cylinder. As you inhale, imagine a plunger forcing the air down to the bottom of the cylinder. The chest (top of the cylinder), does not expand at all; the diaphragm expands to accommodate air. Now, place your hands on your hips level with your navel. Breathe in and feel your abdomen expand out as you keep the shoulders and the chest stable. As you exhale, feel the abdomen fall in toward the body. Next, lay on your back with the hands resting on the abdomen. Concentrate on letting your breath flow into the nostrils as the lower abdomen rises. Breathe out through your mouth as the abdomen descends. Repeat this cycle ten times. This time, breathe in and let the abdomen rise as you visualize oxygen moving into the hands, feet, and head. Breathe out and feel the tension flow out of the body and into the ground beneath you. Try to continue this breathing pattern while you are in the standing position and it will soon become routine.

Three-Part Breathing
Learn to fill up and empty your breath. To begin, sit comfortably in a chair or cross-legged on the floor. Be aware of and feel your sit bones contacting the chair or the floor. Allow your spine to elongate as if a string is gently lifting and pulling the head up. Keep the shoulders and jaw relaxed.

1. Inhale, let your belly fill up with air, and welcome this air into to your body. Allow the belly to get round as it expands away from the body.
2. Let the breath rise into the lungs as you feel expansion around your whole rib cage. Feel the lungs expand from front to back and then from side to side.
3. Bring the breath to the upper chest and allow the collarbones to lengthen and widen away from the center.

4. Shift your attention away from pushing the out air and give attention to yielding your breath to your body. Surrender and relax every muscle, organ, and bone.
5. Exhale and release the air from the upper chest to the middle chest and finally from the abdomen. Your belly will now release towards the spine as the breath transitions for the next in breath.

Start this exercise with a count of four for the in breath and a count of four for the out breath for five minutes, every day. Next, count to six for each breath. Finally, breathe in and out deeply, at a count of eight breaths each. Make the breath feel like the rhythm of a wave flowing through the body. As you relax, you will find that your body will let go on a deeper level. You will notice a pause between each exhalation. Visualize yourself walking upright as you continue to feel the same sensations while you breathe.

Ujjayi breathing

This type of breathing is known as the victory breath. Ujjayi breathing is a diaphragmatic breath that fills the lower belly, rises to the lower ribs, and moves into the upper chest and throat. Inhalation and exhalation are both ultimately done through the nose. It is heard as a hollow, deep, yet soft sound coming from the throat. Ujjayi breath combined with vinyasa makes your movements more fluid and inspiring. You will move as you breathe and breathe as you move. Ujjayi breathing is not difficult to learn. Just relax instead of trying to force the breath.

1. Inhale and exhale all air out of the lungs. On the inhale, pay attention to the sound. It should be smooth and steady. As you inhale, softly whisper the sound "ha" with your mouth open. Stretch the syllable out and feel the air vibrate on the back of the throat. Exhale. Continue for five breaths.
2. Next, close the mouth and make the soft "ha" sound on the inhale and on the exhale. As you exhale, pretend you are fogging up a pair of glasses. It may be easier to make this sound on the exhale. You will breathe through the nostrils with the mouth closed.
3. Make the exhale longer than the inhale and continue for five more breaths. Draw air into the back of the throat as you work through each breath. The rewards of utilizing this type of breathing are to enhance deepening of the breath and strengthening of the diaphragm. The sound in the back of the throat when using Ujjayi breath will help you draw attention to your breath and calm the mind.

Alternate Nostril Breathing

Another yogic breathing exercise is alternate nostril breathing. This technique helps you to build concentration. If you practice it three times a day, you will balance your emotions and increase your lung capacity.

1. Sit in a comfortable position with the head, neck, and spine in alignment.
2. Rest the index and middle finger on the space between the eyebrows. Decide which nostril will be active and which nostril will be passive. The active side will have air flowing through it and the passive side will have an active barrier. You can use the ring finger for the left nostril and your thumb for the right nostril.
3. With one finger, close the passive nostril. Exhale gently through the active nostril and count to six. Then, immediately inhale to a count of six.

4. Now, unblock the passive nostril and close off the active nostril. Exhale through the active nostril and inhale each for a count of six.
5. Repeat this process at least three times. Make each breath smooth and even. When you become more experienced at this technique, increase the length of your breath to a count of eight.

When doing breathing exercises, feel your body expanding on the inhale and contracting on the exhale. Listen to the body and let it tell you what to do. Listen to your breath so that you know how to gauge it and you will know if you need to work harder or if you need to yield. If the breath is labored, back off and if you feel the breath is not flowing swiftly enough, then increase the rate of flow.

If you notice that you are holding your breath, immediately exhale and a natural breath will follow. If you experience discomfort while breathing; inhale into the area of discomfort and exhale the tension out through your feet. Utilize your breath. Your breathing will also remind your client to breathe, in turn, making the pressure and leverage of each technique easier for you to perform.

The environment you work in can have an effect on the way you breathe, how you use your body, and how your posture is. If you work in a confined space, you may have a tendency to breathe in a shallow manner and when you bend over the table, you may round the shoulders, which can constrict breathing by compressing the rib cage. If you are concentrating too hard on the client or a certain technique, you can unknowingly restrict your breath. Restricting space in your body can limit breathing and can be a factor in incorrect usage of your body. You can decrease the demands of your work by breathing correctly and deeply. When you ground and center yourself, bring awareness to the spaciousness within your whole body and your breath. You can give full concentration to your client and still keep some awareness for yourself and your own comfort. This awareness will improve your touch because when you are relaxed and at ease when you work, you will be more connected. When you are more connected, the client will take notice and your touch will feel better. How you express your touch will come from how you feel and how you distinguish yourself in a situation.

Breath is vital. Breath is life. Breath is an essential tool for bodyworkers. Proper breathing helps to keep your energy flowing in the most efficient manner. Breathing deeply gives you increased oxygen and strength. Your mind stays focused if you keep your intention on your breath. You will encourage your client to breathe, if you are breathing deeply. Both your breath and your client's breath will become synchronized as the massage is performed. Your energy level will not diminish as quickly if you continue full, deep breathing throughout the entire massage. Paying attention to your body includes paying attention to your breath. Notice if you are holding your breath and resume breathing. The concept of breath awareness will keep oxygen flowing through your body during the entire massage. Proper breathing brings you into your body and out of your mind, which will bring grace and fluidity to each of your movements.

Breath is the barometer for your energy and your emotions. It is the base for the attentiveness of your body and your emotions. Most people pay a small amount of attention to their breath, yet without your breath, you could not survive. It takes only a small amount of time to become skilled in proper breathing. Proper breathing will activate important energy centers in your body and it can improve many aspects of your life. Pay attention and think of a how a sleeping baby breathes next time you are not properly breathing. When a baby is breathing, the belly will swell and release, as the hips and shoulders rock, and the spine ripples. Allow your whole body to breathe, give the muscles and organs a mini-massage as it soothes and calms every cell in the body.

Tips to remember for proper breathing:

- How you think and feel can affect breathing.
- Remember that the breath and posture are interrelated.
- Breath is movement.
- Correct breathing is about proper inhalation and exhalation.
- Deep breathing can increase the amount and percent of oxygen you take in.
- Move your belly with your breath and keep the upper body quiet.
- Let your belly fill up on the inhale before the lungs expand with air.
- Let the air flow out from top, to middle, to bottom of the chest to empty air out on the exhale.
- Keep your breath moving evenly as you concentrate on your work.
- Lengthen the exhalations and pause after each exhalation.
- Allow the whole body to breathe.

Chapter Fifteen

Yoga

The practice of yoga originated in India. The word yoga translates as union. This union is of the body, mind, and spirit. For thousands of years, yoga has been a tool to open the mind and body to bring transformation and self-awareness.

The physical body tightens as you live daily life, exercise, and age. As your body becomes less flexible and more stiff, it becomes less efficient and more prone to injury and disease. Physically, if you are tight, you become internally constricted. Yoga helps by lessening the constriction of bodily tissues and can help to slow, and even reverse the aging process.

Many people think that yoga is simply stretching. Stretching is included but yoga creates balance by developing strength and flexibility in the body. The way of achieving this balance is through a series of postures or poses called asanas. Each pose has a particular physical benefit. The poses can be done in either a fast or slow pace. The fast paced, steady rhythm helps to create heat in the body. The slow, flowing pace is done to perfect the alignment of each pose, increase stamina, and release each stretch point in the tissue. The postures are done in succession, but the approach depends on what tradition is being taught.

Many physical benefits come from a regular yoga practice. Three main benefits of yoga are increased strength, flexibility, and better balance. When you feel energetic and strong, you feel light. When you feel tired and weak, you feel extremely heavy. A steady yoga practice will make you feel stronger and lighter and give better tone to your muscles. Doing yoga erases the muscle tension in your body. With a regular yoga practice, your body becomes more fluid, moves more efficiently, and increases flexibility. Consequently, pain and tension are less likely to be stored in the body. Yoga creates symmetry in your body and makes you strong and flexible, in a balanced manner. As a result, balance seems to happen in all areas of your life.

Yoga gives strength and flexibility for physical activity, and on a deeper level, yoga generates energy. The energy yoga brings has a more focused quality. Practicing yoga will keep you in the present moment and help with your body awareness. The art of yoga allows you to accept your limits, and listen to and honor your body. It also teaches you how to balance many aspects of your life.

Yoga helps to train your mind in a more concentrated way and helps to keep the mind focused. It brings mental clarity and increased peace of mind. Yoga gives feedback from the physical body to the mind, allowing awareness to be transferred when practicing bodywork. The body has its own built in intelligence. You will learn to listen to the intelligence of your own body through the practice of yoga. A great side effect from practicing yoga is learning to focus your energy. Through yoga, you will cultivate feedback sensitivity. You will learn to feel the difference between pain and intensity. This concept will allow a sense of awareness and counter tendencies to ignore the body's feedback messages. Pain is feedback. Notice and make a mental note of slight pains or twinges. Also, observe any feelings of numbness or tingling. Any sensations that are felt, if only for a second, need to be paid attention to and noted. This serves as a warning to you.

To practice yoga, wear loose and comfortable clothing. A non-slip surface or mat is essential. A folding chair and a pillow need to be kept to the side. A blanket and a strap are also very useful for modifying different poses. A quiet, undisturbed place is very important for focusing the mind. The most important thing you need to bring to your mat is a big heart and a small ego. The best time for yoga is in the morning before breakfast, but it can be done anytime. It is preferred to practice yoga on an empty stomach. Always start with easy poses for warm-up and then progress to more difficult poses. Rest at the end of every yoga practice to integrate yourself back into reality.

The building blocks of a yoga practice are comprised of seven different movements. Every posture is a combination of one of the seven movements. The movements are flexion, extension, hyperextension, abduction, adduction, rotation, and circumduction. Postures are to be done gradually to release tight and constricted areas. Your yoga practice is to be used for self-observation and self-healing. Yoga is not a competition, nor is it a destination. Awareness is one of the most important aspects of your practice.

Proper breathing brings life to a pose. Synchronize your movements with your breath. Some movements begin on the inhale and some on the exhale. Movements that are expansive and opening, such as backbends and open arms, begin on an inhale. Contracting and closing postures, such as a forward bend, start with an exhale. The type of breath you use depends on what happens naturally for your body. Let your body guide you from within. Yoga helps you to concentrate and live in the now. Using the breath and flowing with each posture will improve your ability to feel, listen, and concentrate on yourself.

Breath and movement should become one. Link breath and movement, breathe without restrictions, inhale on expansion and exhale with contracting or folding poses, and let the breath guide you. Feel yourself as you move with angel arms. Breathe and inhale as you raise your arms to the sides and above the head. Exhale and allow the arms to return down to the sides of the body. Include smoothness, depth, and steadiness in your breathing. Let the breath bring the poses to life as you express your individuality and enhance your life.

It is a good idea to start the session seated to center yourself and to collect energy. Think of what your intention or purpose for the session is. A seated, cross-legged position is a common way to start your session. The next step in the session is to warm up. You can do the warm up phase seated or standing. The warm up phase focuses on the breath and increases flexibility in the connective tissue and joints. Another common way to warm up is to stand and flow through the sun salutation three times. Standing poses help to align your body and bring awareness to each posture. Tadasana or mountain pose is a great way to start standing poses. It is one of the most basic poses and the foundation for standing postures. Stand with your feet hip width apart and your arms at your side. Feel the ground under your feet. Bring your pelvis to neutral and feel your body lift from the bottom of the spine through the top of the head. Fix your gaze at a specific place in front of you. Breathe smoothly, relax, and be in the stillness.

The benefits of standing poses are to create a firm foundation through the feet and legs, develop strength, flexibility, balance, and emphasize stabilization for the spine. Twists can be added for decompressing the spine, massaging internal organs, and relaxing the central nervous system. Some examples of a twist are sage twist, seated spinal twist, and crocodile twist. Seated postures promote flexibility of the arms and back; they balance the energizing effects of standing postures and create a foundation at the pelvis. Some examples of a seated posture are bound angle, half forward bend, and full forward bend. Inversions like downward facing dog, bridge, and plow are helpful to open the shoulders. Inversions are useful for reversing the effects of gravity, increasing circulation, and strengthening the immune system. The next step in sequencing is to release the spine and prepare for relaxation. Releases help to ease the spine of tension, prepare for relaxation, and slow the breath down. Pelvic tilt and knees to chest pose are great examples of a release. Savasana is the final relaxation pose and is actually the goal of yoga. This pose may be the most challenging of all poses because you have to just "be". You have to be in the present moment and let go of all thoughts. In other words, just be with the quiet and stillness. Savasana or corpse pose completes the session with renewed energy. This final step leads to relaxation and should be done seated in locust pose or laying face up in corpse pose.

An important aspect of Yoga is that it teaches you lines of energy. Lines of energy are currents that move in certain directions, in particular postures. You will start to notice that some parts of your body feel vital and strong, while some parts feel weak and blocked. Learning to feel these lines of energy while you work will create alignment. This alignment will, in turn, create strength.

Triangle pose creates five lines of energy. (15.1) In triangle pose, you have one line of energy from your shoulder to the raised arm up through the fingertips. This line opens the chest and allows the pelvis to align. Second, the energy moves from the hip down the back of the leg to the foot and raises the arch. The second line frees the hip and aligns the pelvis. Then, the energy moves from the hip, down the front leg to the foot. This action lines up the knee with the pelvis. Next, the energy moves up the spine allowing space between the vertebrae as it unlocks the hip. Finally, a line moves from the shoulder down to the fingertips on the lower arm. This movement creates alignment from the shoulder to the pelvis and gives your posture greater depth.

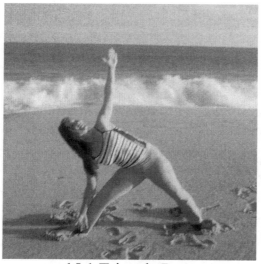

15.1 Triangle Pose

When using this dimension of energy you automatically align yourself from the inside out. You are allowed to feel and sense where you are in your own space. When alignment is felt internally, the body uses its own intelligence and the posture is understood completely.

Yoga adds additional benefits to the bodyworker and is an excellent cross-training resistance workout. Using your own body's resistance will create core strength, better balance, and coordination. Deep and relaxed breathing exercises the lungs and teaches you how to breathe correctly. Yoga increases flexibility and range of motion while relieving muscle tension. Yoga also helps you to feel your body kinesthetically from the inside out.

Yoga can be practiced safely and can be a great addition to your fitness routine. Yoga is generally safe when performed correctly and if taught by an experienced instructor. If you begin practicing yoga with a qualified instructor you can prevent injuries, figure out your limitations, and learn how to listen to your body. In the beginning, it is important to start slowly and learn the fundamentals first. Move through the postures slowly and carefully, especially when beginning a yoga practice. If the class is not right for you or your teacher is pushing you too far and not helping with modifications then switch classes. Videotapes at home are a good method, but I like to see students go to classes and be observed. A teacher can offer modifications and adjustments that you will not get on your own at home. The most common injuries that happen in yoga are created by repetitive stress or overstretching. These injuries occur at the neck, shoulders, wrists, at the sacroiliac joint, along the spine, knees, and hamstrings.

Most new students of yoga are young, healthy, and competitive. Students push themselves too far and ignore their edge. They go into positions that they are not experienced in and strain their muscles or pull a ligament. The body will only stretch to the point it is set at. Flexibility and muscle strength take time to develop and the body will adjust, but it takes time and patience. Remember that yoga is not competitive. Concentrate only on what is going on within your own body and be in the present moment. It does not matter how far your neighbor is going into a certain posture. Focus on your breath and your own body. You are unique and your goals are as well. You are in a process of self-discovery. This is why it is a good idea to cross-train when you are involved in a bodywork career. It makes you live in the present moment and stay grounded as you pay attention to your body from the inside out.

The shoulders are an integral link from your hands to your body. Shoulder injuries or instability can be common for the manual therapist. Yoga can be very beneficial for the shoulders, but it can also cause harm if not practiced correctly. When you use yoga to create strength and stability, make sure you build strength correctly without causing or aggravating an injury. To prevent injuries, analyze your shoulders in every pose and maintain proper alignment. If you have a shoulder injury, modify poses and avoid all weight bearing such as downward facing dog, plank, or chattaranga (four-limbed staff pose). Also, approach shoulder openers with caution.

Joint instability, impingements, rotator cuff strains or tears, and arthritis are common injuries. Shoulders are designed for mobility, not stability. This mobility permits a wide range of motion. If your shoulders are healthy, you can move the arm front, back, across the body, and in 360 degree circles. If the joint is loose and unstable, the soft tissue has to hold it together which can place it more at risk for injury. The ball and socket joint is situated in a shallow manner in the shoulder joint.

140

Visualize a softball on top of a plunger. The softball is the head of the humerus and the plunger is where it meets the scapula. The shoulder is mobile because of the big ball on a small base. When the soft tissue surrounding the joint is strong and toned, everything works impeccably. In contrast, repetitive movements can cause problems in the muscles around the joint and the ligaments can overstretch and lose elasticity. Also, as muscles age they tend to lose tone and can create instability for the joint. The best way to keep stability around the joint is to build balanced strength around it.

To build strength in the shoulder joint, perfect alignment is essential. Poor posture is habitual and can be hard to break if you are not mindful. Yoga can help you be mindful and keep the shoulders from slumping or internally rotating. Misalignments should be noticed during your daily life and not carried into your yoga practice. When practicing yoga, widen the collarbones to prevent the shoulders from rounding or internally rotating and make sure the upper back is engaged by drawing the shoulder blades down and together. These movements help to protect the back of the shoulder joints. If practiced often, these shoulder movements will eventually become an integral part of your practice.

Check your alignment frequently. The risk of shoulder injury is increased dramatically in weight bearing yoga if misalignments are present. Explore yourself in Tadasana (standing mountain pose). First, lift your shoulders so they are in line with the base of the neck and draw the heads of the arm bones back toward the wall behind you. Keep the natural curve in your neck and draw the shoulder blades down your back. Keep the tips of the shoulder blades pressing into the back and spreading. Now try reaching the arms overhead. Rotate the arm bones externally and move the head of the bone into the socket. The external rotation of the shoulder strengthens the infraspinatus and teres minor as it saves the supraspinatus from injury. Once you lift the arms overhead, reach upward and spread the shoulder blades away from each other. Feel the shoulder blades wrap around toward the front of the rib cage and lengthen up as you create more space. The shoulders should lift slightly as you press the palms toward the ceiling. These movements are comparable to handstand, only a handstand is upside down and weight-bearing.

After proper alignment is learned, it is time for strength to be built and maintained. Done correctly, yoga poses strengthen the shoulders. However, the shoulders have to be strong to perform the poses correctly and maintain proper alignment. For example, in chaturanga or four limbed staff pose, if the shoulders are not strong enough to be held in the proper place, you are more susceptible to injury. In this pose, you are either on all fours or in a push up position. If the chest collapses in chaturanga, the head of the arm bones will drop toward the floor. The shoulder blades will then slide out instead of lying flat against the back. If you do not set yourself in the correct alignment in this pose, the front of your shoulders will be sore the next day. This can strain the front of the rotator cuff and build strength unequally. It makes the front of the rotator cuff stronger than the rear. To offset this misalignment, start in plank pose (push up position) and move your body to the floor in chaturanga. Make sure that the head of the arm bones stay level with the elbows. Do not let them drop. Build strength around the whole rotator cuff. You can start with your knees on the floor until ample strength is built. Also, reverse plank in the face up position can strengthen certain muscles as it stretches the opposing muscles worked in chaturanga. Stretching the front of the chest with camel (15.2), bridge pose, fish pose, and shoulderstand, in correct alignment, can create balance and additional flexibility.

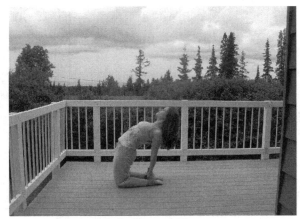
15.2 Camel Pose

To create more stability in the shoulder joint, it is also a good idea to concentrate on the supraspinatus. This muscle initiates the action of raising the shoulder to the side and lifting it from shoulder height to above the head. To strengthen the supraspinatus, perform standing postures with the arms reaching out. Some examples for strengthening the supraspinatus are triangle pose and warrior II. Once the shoulder joint is stable and pain free, then weight-bearing postures can be added. A great way to build strength in the rotator cuff is to slowly move from downward facing dog to chaturanga and back again. Be mindful not to let the upper back hyperextend and sink toward the floor in downward facing dog. As you move into plank, maintain width in the upper back to keep the shoulder girdle active and shoulder joints stable. In yoga, many poses build arm strength by pushing away from the floor. Poses like downward facing dog (15.3), shoulderstand, and upward facing bow, require you to push against the floor. Few poses necessitate the shoulder muscles to pull against resistance and the result is that the rotator muscles in the back of the shoulders get weak. A way to build strength in the back of the shoulder is to perform movements that require pulling, like swimming or pull-ups. Also, do exercises that press the back of the shoulders against the floor. An example of opening the shoulders would be bridge pose with the palms flat on the floor.

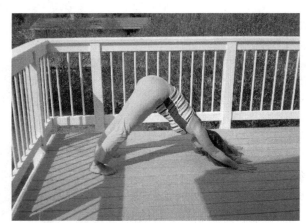
15.3 Downward Facing Dog Pose

Finally, to generate balanced flexibility, practice poses that require inward rotation of the shoulder. Examples of postures that involve inward rotation are cow face pose, marichi's twist III and side stretch pose. Avoid inward rotation if you feel a pinching sensation or have a history of dislocation or shoulder instability.

The wrist is one of the initial joints in the kinetic chain. The wrist can carry a lot of tension and be injured easily if too much strain is placed on it. Wrist pain can be caused by a variety of reasons. Wrist pain can be a result of tense flexor muscles in the forearm, tight tendons in the wrist, trauma, cysts, anatomical changes in the wrist, or specific syndromes like carpal tunnel. If your wrists are currently injured, avoid weight-bearing poses with the hands. If the pain and inflammation has subsided, the use of props can help to modify poses and prevent further injury. The use of a foam wedge can decrease the angle of extension of the wrist in such poses as upward and downward facing dog as well as, some arm balances. Also, modifications can be taught to avoid putting pressure on the wrist joint. For example, in downward facing dog you can substitute dolphin pose and for plank pose you can substitute forearm plank using the forearms on the floor instead of the wrists. Another modification that can be done at the wall is right angle posture where the arms and torso are parallel to the floor and no pressure is on the wrist itself. All of these ideas help to diminish the pressure of your body weight on the wrist joints.

If poses are practiced correctly, the shoulders, wrists, and the rest of your body will remain injury-free. There are no guarantees in yoga or in life. Pain is your body's way of asking you to listen and examine what you are doing. If injuries do occur, remember that injuries can be a wonderful blessing, as they offer us an opportunity to learn, grow, and help others.

When yoga students have limitations because of an injury, internal conflict can arise since poses have to be modified. Doing something different can create reluctance. However, if you practice contentment, you will learn to accept what is in the present moment and not struggle with how your body is supposed to be functioning. This type of acceptance can lead you chose the appropriate pose and allow your injury to heal.

Your specific anatomy and health history are unique and need to be factored in when you decide which type of yoga is for you. Study each type of yoga, decide what your goals are and choose which style is best for creating balance in your life. Yoga can be done by yourself and is called your personal practice, or it can be in a classroom setting. Each tradition varies and there are different styles for every person. In your personal practice, your individual experience with yoga develops over time as you learn to listen to your body and quiet your mind. In a classroom setting you can receive modifications and adjustments from your teacher to refine your alignment. The styles of yoga range from flowing, to active, slow, or restorative. Yoga definitely offers something for everyone!

Demystifying yoga seems difficult, but if you know what your body's needs are and you educate yourself, it is pretty simple. Yoga classes are offered for beginners, intermediate, and advanced students. If you are new to yoga then definitely take a beginners class and learn the fundamentals. From that point, you can branch off into whichever specialty you would like.

Various yogis from India have developed different types of yoga. Some are done gently and some are vigorous and fast paced. Restorative yoga is more passive, and helps the body to heal and the mind to relax. Poses are generally held for several minutes. Props such as bolsters and blankets are used to support you in each posture. Holding poses for an extended period of time allows the muscles to relax and gravity to work. Restorative yoga is easy and is great for stressed out people, pregnant, or overweight students. Also, restorative yoga helps chronic conditions such as fibromyalgia, migraines, and back problems.

Kripalu yoga is tranquil yoga and is based on compassion. Kripalu means to breathe, relax, feel, watch, and allow. The student moves at their own pace, honors the body's needs, and explores the emotions in each pose. You can practice light, easy stretching in this class or gentle, flowing poses that emphasize thoughts, feelings, and emotions. These classes are great for stress-relief, pregnant, postpartum, and beginner students.

Kundalini yoga helps your life force energy flow and balances the chakras. Kundalini is gentle, yet invigorating. Movements are dynamic with rocking and twisting. Active exercises are followed by deep relaxation, meditation, or chanting. Kundalini is gentle yet invigorating and is great for beginners and anyone with an open mind.

Scaravelli yoga is a precise type of yoga with a soft and fluid method. Unwinding and relaxing the body are the goals with this type of yoga. Scaravelli put emphasis on aligning the spine and is excellent for students of any age and any level.

Viniyoga matches your practice with your basic needs. Viniyoga is often called therapeutic yoga and uses the breath to flow with the movement. You can practice in a class or, if you have a specific need, you can hire a personal instructor. Viniyoga can suit anyone from an athlete to one with a chronic illness. This type of yoga is a flowing, moving meditation.

Iyengar yoga pays attention to the muscular and skeletal alignment in each pose. Alignment is essential for free flowing energy. Props are widely used in Iyengar yoga to ensure alignment and assist flexibility. Iyengar can be difficult because of the strict emphasis on alignment, but it can be very insightful for your daily practice.

Bikram yoga loosens and relaxes your muscles in a hot room for nearly ninety minutes. You are led through twenty-six hatha yoga postures, twice. Total body benefits, cardio conditioning, and toxin release are included in this class. Consistency of workout is a benefit of Bikram. One class fits all and this class is not for beginners. This is a challenging type of yoga but you will leave the class with a sense of lightness and freedom.

Power yoga is a blend of Ashtanga, Bikram, and Iyengar. Power yoga is a fitness-based, vinyasa style approach. It mixes strength, flexibility, and agility. Power yoga also includes breathwork and a minimal amount of chanting. Power yoga is a blend and does not follow a set series of postures. Power yoga is a great workout, but you may not get the individual attention if you are a beginner. The pace is fast and the mixture of types is powerful. You will find this type of yoga in many American gyms.

Active restorative yoga is taught with a lot of inversions and provides you with energy. Inverted poses rejuvenate the body from the inside out, develop upper body strength, and reduce effects of gravity on the spine. The nervous system is strengthened and the endocrine system is stimulated. Headstand and shoulderstand are reviving inversions that should only be taught by a teacher. Students with high blood pressure, neck or shoulder injuries, glaucoma, or women who are pregnant or menstruating should avoid inversions. Active restorative yoga gives great energy and fresh oxygen to the brain.

Ashtanga yoga is for the mind, body, and spirit, and is the perfect workout for someone who wants a challenge. Originally, Ashtanga yoga was developed with a blend of yoga, gymnastics, and Indian wrestling. This type of yoga uses breathwork as it conditions, strengthens, and stretches the body. A blend of sun salutations, inversions, and balancing poses are taught in this version of yoga. This class is for more advanced students and is excellent for a vigorous and challenging workout.

Regardless of your size, religion, or athleticism, yoga can offer better strength, balance, cardiovascular health, flexibility, and stronger bones. Yoga offers many physical and mental benefits to each person. Increased body awareness will give you greater self-confidence and insight for your body. The stress-reducing qualities of yoga are priceless and can help you to live a happier and healthier life. There are many types of yoga that can suit each person's individual needs. Find one that is right for you and allow yoga to enhance your life.

Points to remember with yoga:

- Your physical body can benefit greatly from practicing yoga.
- Yoga can help with your alignment and awareness in bodywork.
- Yoga helps to keep the mind focused.
- Yoga is a great cross-training workout for bodyworkers.
- Yoga links breath and movement.
- Yoga gives your body added strength and flexibility.
- There are many types of yoga that can be practiced for every need and ability.
- Yoga links mind, body, and spirit.

Chapter Sixteen

Traditional Chinese Exercises

Throughout history every culture has recognized the presence of some type of life force energy in the human body. In western culture, we refer to life force energy as human electricity. In India, energy is called Prana, in China it is Chi, and in Japan it is referred to as Ki. In the east and the west, energy is perceived as an animating life force that allows you to attain certain physical goals and maintain good health. Chinese exercises have been a tradition for over 2500 years. Chinese methods have come to the U.S. and have helped to prolong health and retain longevity of people's lives. Research has demonstrated the effectiveness of these therapeutic exercises to the physiological system.

Traditional Chinese Medicine thinks of energy as Chi and knows that an unrestricted flow of Chi through the energy pathways is essential for good health. Chi is an electromagnetic energy that runs through your body and it affects everything that you do. The more Chi that is moving freely throughout your body, the more energetic and active you will feel.

Chinese exercises combine slow and gentle movements with mental concentration. As a result of performing these exercises, the heart, muscles, and lungs are strengthened. Emotional and psychological states are improved as balance and a sense of harmony occur between the body and mind. Chinese exercises improve physical fitness and are gentle enough for the elderly. These movements can correct posture, increase blood circulation, assist with flexibility, and calm the body and mind. Chinese exercises can improve posture, body awareness, and help improve flexibility of the joints and the spine for bodyworkers. These methods can also help the energy system stay clear and flow freely.

There are various Chinese exercises that you can do to keep your energy flowing and maintain your health. The exercises suggested for the bodyworker include: Tai Chi, Chi Kung, and Ba Duan Jin. All exercises should be used in combination with slow breathing. Most of the movements are symbolic so try to imagine what each represents for you as you do each exercise. Begin each exercise by visualizing yourself protected by a cocoon of golden light. Start and end the exercises by gathering and storing Chi in your lower Dan Tien. These exercises can be practiced any time, but sunrise is the best time of day to practice. The various exercises are best practiced in loose clothes, barefoot in the grass and close to a tree. How long you practice depends on your health and enthusiasm. Beginners can start with 15 minutes every morning and every evening. Intermediate people can practice these exercises for 30 minutes two times a day and advanced people can practice as long as they feel comfortable.

Tai Chi Chuan is an ancient martial art and its foundation comes from Taoist philosophy. Tai Chi is an exercise of great origin that uses the hands and the body to perform slow, fluid movements. This exercise combines yin and yang in a balanced way and is gentle and relaxing. It is comparable to a form of moderate exercise. It has great advantages for all ages and many different types of illnesses. Those with arthritis and high blood pressure can benefit greatly from Tai Chi. Each exercise moves the muscles and joints in the limbs of your body. Executing the movements require relaxation of the muscles of the wrists, arms, shoulders, chest, abdomen, and back. It is important to keep all of the joints open so Chi can flow through the body uninterrupted. The limbs should move more effortlessly as coordination and balance are improved through the use of Tai Chi. Each movement of Tai Chi is executed by thought and energy, rather than strength. Concentrating on the movements is very important to relaxing the mind and focusing your concentration. Remember that Tai Chi is also a breathing exercise.

Tai Chi is done with meticulous, repetitive movements and with the body upright and relaxed. The practice of Tai Chi is 173 movements in all. The short or yin form can be practiced or you can perform the long or yang form. You must first learn Tai Chi from an experienced teacher. After being instructed on the correct form, you will be able to practice Tai Chi on your own.

It is important to start with the basics. Begin with the basic martial arts stance to gain energy and become grounded. Stand with your feet shoulder width apart and the toes pointed forward. Keep the knees and elbows slightly bent as your arms extend slightly out from your body. Leave some space under the armpit and feel your hands becoming heavy and relaxed. Keep the spine straight as your eyes gaze softly forward and concentrate your weight into your feet as you sink slightly down towards the floor. Feel your body pressing down until you are anchored into the earth. Allow your breath to flow up your back, around the top of the head, and down the front of your body in a circular fashion. Hold this position for three to five minutes. After some time of practicing this stance, you will build strength in the legs and center your mind as you let energy flow throughout your entire body. After time, you will be able to sink more weight down into your legs as you learn how to relax.

Chi Kung, also known as Qi Gong, is a breath training and invigorating exercise. It merges breathing with meditation and exercise. Chi Kung is a way of accumulating life energy through exercise. Chi Kung includes adjustments of your mind, breath, and posture. Chi Kung is useful in preserving the energy of the body. This is why Chi Kung is very important for the bodyworker because it is an energy building exercise.

Most everyone can benefit from Chi Kung energy work. To practice Chi Kung, you need to relax the body and mind as you focus your attention and breathe evenly. The training of concentration and breath is very helpful for every bodyworker. Chi Kung is an art and a skill. Patience and gradual development are the keys to success. The length of the practice is up to the practitioner, but is most commonly done for 15-45 minutes. Start by counting your breaths with one breath counting as an inhale and an exhale. Count from one to ten breaths and follow your breath with your attention. After a couple of weeks of practicing Chi Kung, concentrate your breath into your lower abdomen. Once you feel you have gotten this down, follow your breath on an inhale from your nose to the lungs and on the exhale feel the breath flow from the lungs to your nose. If thoughts distract you, bring yourself back to your breath. Continue breathing in this circular fashion while doing each exercise.

Chi Kung is a method of building and balancing energy through exercise. The three keys to regulating the body are postural alignment, relaxation, and building strong roots for grounding. Postural alignment is important because Chi will not flow through an area that contains tension. Relaxation is a very important principle to Chi Kung because when you relax the body the bones move easier, which allows chi to flow easier. Building strong roots for grounding means you will have a secure contact with your feet touching the ground. Grounding helps you to maintain a strong foundation for your whole body.

The exercise Standing like a Tree puts emphasis on these three principles. (16.1) To feel rooted into the ground, stand with your feet hip width apart with the legs, pelvis, spine, head, and neck vertically aligned. Your shoulders will remain relaxed with the arms in front of you like they are wrapping around a tree. Let the arms and fingers relax as they hold this position. Relax into your core and breathe into your Dan Tien by taking slow, deep breaths. Your hips and buttocks will stay relaxed while the knees are soft and slightly bent. Let your weight be evenly distributed between both feet. Feel roots penetrating deep into the earth from your feet. Below your knees, feel your root system flow downward to draw earth energy up from the ground. Above the knees, visualize yourself growing like a tree so you can draw in the heaven energy from above. Practice mindfulness when doing this exercise while breathing deeply and evenly. This exercise allows you to feel a confident contact with the ground and a foundation of support for the whole body.

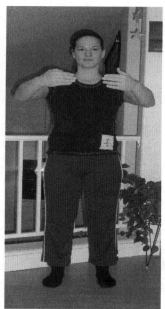

16.1 Standing like A Tree

Ba Duan Jin consists of eight standing exercises. It is a type of medical Qi Gong designed to improve health. The name of each exercise illustrates each movement and its outcome on the body. Effort is exerted with this exercise but most of the effort is internal. It regulates the internal organs and relieves fatigue. Ba Duan Jin is very successful in strengthening your arm, leg, and chest muscles and helps to improve your posture. With this exercise, you will inhale on the stretch and exhale on the release. Feel the breath moving up into the body on the inhale and let all tension flow out of your body on the exhale. Generally, Ba Duan Jin is a more invigorating exercise but it can be practiced slowly and more gently for elderly or ill patients.

Other Chinese exercises can be done to improve health, flexibility, and posture. You, as a bodyworker, can achieve great benefits from doing these exercises. The Dan Tien is located two inches below the umbilicus. Stroking the Dan Tien can help any abdominal discomfort and help to build an energy reserve in this area. Massage this point with three fingers of the right hand for around five minutes. Also, stroking the Yung Chuan is helpful for grounding. The Yung Chuan is located below the ball of the foot in the middle. This point is good for strengthening the feet. Start with stroking the left foot with three fingers of the right hand until you feel warmth. Another useful exercise is to swing the arms because it is good to keep the shoulder joints in shape and flexible. Stand with the feet shoulder width apart with your arms at the side. Swing both arms forward and upward to navel height. Switch to swinging your arms rhythmically downward and backward. Continue swinging your arms with your pelvis swaying the same way your arms are moving. Repeat this motion one to two hundred times while remaining as relaxed as possible. Keep your breath flowing throughout this exercise.

The exercise, riding a horse, can be useful to strengthen the quadriceps and knees. (16.2) Stand with feet forward and more than hip width apart. The spine will be tall and your elbows will be bent at the sides with the hands made into a soft fist. Bend the knees like you are riding a horse and hold this position for two to three minutes. Return to the starting position and then bend the knees for three more minutes while you bend and straighten the arms out in front of you. Breathe deeply while you are performing this exercise. Last, stand with shoulders hip width apart with toes pointed slightly out. Bend your knees to around 90 degrees and rest the hands on the thighs. Keep the chest open and the body centered. Do some deep breathing exercises and hold this position as long as possible.

Chinese exercises will help your energy flow and keep you in a vibrant state of health. The human body is constantly vibrating with energy and this energy needs to be balanced and kept flowing freely. Overall physical and mental health is a byproduct of free flowing energy. When the meridians or the energy field is out of sync or the energy is disturbed, illness can result. Chinese exercises combined with western exercises can be of great benefit to the health of all of the body systems, particularly the physical.

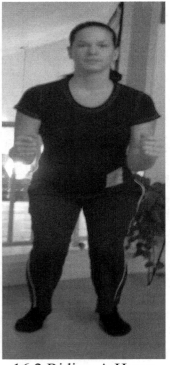

16.2 Riding A Horse

It is necessary for you to carry out physical exercises to keep up with the rigorous demands you place on your body. Bodywork calls for physical strength and stamina because you may hold positions for certain periods of time. Doing a variety of exercises will keep you fit and prepare you for your work. Chinese exercises will also help you to build up your energy reserve and assist you with the healing of your client without depleting your own energy reserve.

Traditional Chinese Exercises assist with:

- Posture
- Blood circulation
- Flexibility
- Calming the mind and body
- Chi circulation
- Body awareness
- Joint mobility
- Breathing
- Concentration

Chapter Seventeen

Nutrition

To sustain your health and energy as a bodyworker, you must remember to eat properly. You need to think of yourself as an athlete and fuel your body as an athlete would. Your body does physical activity for many hours a day and nutrition should be very important to you. You are what you eat and you want your body to utilize nutrients in the most efficient manner.

The energy source your body depends on is obtained from nutrients. Food energy provides nutrients and creates energy for the maintenance of your health and the immune system of the body. Nutrition is the sum total of processes involved in the intake and utilization of food substances by living organisms including ingestion, digestion, absorption, transport, and metabolism of nutrients found in food. The primary purpose of eating is to provide your body with a variety of nutrients. Major nutrients serve three basic functions. The first function of nutrients is for energy provision. Carbohydrates and fats are the primary sources of energy. The second function is to promote growth and development by building and repairing the body's tissues. Protein is the major building material for muscles and other soft tissues. Therefore, protein is very important in rebuilding your muscle tissue after breaking it down. Last, nutrients are used to help regulate metabolism. For your body to function efficiently you need over 40 essential nutrients in specific amounts. Hippocrates acknowledged that food must be your medicine and medicine must be your food. What you eat plays an important role in the development or progression of a variety of diseases.

A balanced intake of carbohydrates, fats, protein, vitamins, minerals, and water are necessary for proper performance. The three keys to maintaining a healthy diet would include: variety, balance, and moderation. A balanced proportion of food from all different food groups is recommended. Remember, you are what you eat. Select whole, natural foods that will provide the proper amount of nutrients for optimal functioning.

You should obtain nutrients from a variety of unprocessed, whole foods. Consume only the amount of calories you expend daily to regulate body weight. Be sure to include essential fatty acids in your diet. Flax seed and fish oil are excellent sources of these fatty acids. Eat less high fat meat and more fish. Fish contain omega-3, an essential fatty acid. Eat white-fleshed fish such as cod, sole, halibut, and sea bass. These types of fish are easy to digest and nourish the body's organs, muscles, tendons, and bones. Eat meat that is organically raised and eat dairy products that are low in fat. Avoid additives and buy foods that are fresh and organic. Fresh foods are recommended because canned or packages foods contain artificial flavors, colors and preservatives. Fresh food also contains more active Chi. Foods that are high in saturated fat, such as high fat meat, full fat dairy products, baked goods, or commercially prepared foods should be kept to a minimum. Limit your intake of fast foods because these products are generally high in fat. Most fast food sandwiches derive 50 percent of their calories from fat. When cooking, try to boil or bake your foods instead of frying.

Generally speaking, 50 to 60 percent of your calories should come from carbohydrates. Choose more complex carbohydrates and smaller amounts of simple carbohydrates. Focus on whole grains, legumes, fruits, and vegetables. Eat raw fruits and vegetables whenever possible, especially ones high in beta-carotene and vitamin C. Some examples of foods containing vitamin C are citrus fruits, strawberries, peppers, and kiwis. Some examples of Beta-carotene are carrots, peaches, squash, sweet potatoes, and dark, leafy greens. Also, increase your intake of cruciferous vegetables such as cabbage, broccoli, cauliflower, and brussel sprouts. Aim for three to five servings of fruits and vegetables a day.

Sugar is sweet but is it good for you to eat? Sugar can suppress the immune system, contribute to asthma and arthritis, and lead to hypertension. Sugar has many detrimental effects on the body so it is best used in moderation. Make an effort to decrease your intake levels of refined sugars. Check food labels to see if sugar is one of the first listed and if this is the case, avoid the product. Try using naturally occurring sugars to satisfy your needs.

Maintain your intake of protein at adequate and moderate levels. Most of the protein Americans consume is from animal sources. Plant proteins are better since they are lower in saturated fat. Protein is used as an energy source under certain conditions. Three to six ounces of meat, fish, and poultry as well as, two glasses of skim or soymilk, contains the Recommended Dietary Allowance (RDA) for protein. Carbohydrates are the main source of energy for endurance athletes. Consuming adequate amounts of carbohydrates will lessen the utilization of protein during exercise and maintain normal protein stores in the body. The timing of protein intake is important. It is believed that supplying your body with protein within an hour following exercise assists in the repair and rebuilding of muscle tissue. More blood flow to the muscle during recovery allows more amino acids to be delivered to the tissues.

Proper fluid replacement is very important to your body's hydration. Water provides no food energy but constitutes a lot of your body weight and helps nutrients to function. The amount of water needed varies by the weight of the individual. The average adult needs two to three quarts of water a day. Proper water and electrolyte balance is very important for the bodyworker. Water helps to protect the body tissues, especially the brain and spinal cord. Water is the main component of blood and is valuable in the functioning of all your senses. It flushes toxins from the organs and helps to aid in the control of weight.

The diet you intake is effective in regulating your weight, especially if done in combination with cardiovascular exercise. Cardiovascular exercise helps to increase blood flow and reduces the risk of carpal tunnel syndrome in bodyworkers because it increases circulation to the tissues. The key for weight loss is selecting low-calorie, high-nutrient foods.

Enjoy your food. Eat whole fruit whenever possible. If whole fruits are not available, try to drink fruit juice that is 100 percent fruit juice. Buy bread products that list whole wheat as the first ingredient. Keep raw fruits, vegetables, and nuts around for snacks. Before performing a massage, you should intake a sufficient amount of fluid, foods high in complex carbohydrates, and a moderate amount of protein. A balanced breakfast is very important to start your day.

Examples of a serving of complex carbohydrates include:

- One half of a cup of whole grain cereal, grains, or pasta
- One slice of whole grain bread
- One whole grain waffle
- One small baked potato, sweet potato, or a half cup of squash
- Two brown rice cakes

Good nutrition is essential to your body, especially if you have an imbalance, ailment, or an injury. Supplementation can help with arthritis, tendonitis, and muscle soreness. Supplementation such as Methylsulfonylmethane (MSM), flax oil, or fish oil can be helpful when dealing with arthritis. Omega-3 and omega-6 fatty acids are important to include in your diet. The omega-3 fatty acids are found in fish oil and the omega-6 are found in seed and vegetable oils. A great source of omega-6 is borage oil and is outstanding as an anti-inflammatory. Impaired absorption can sometimes occur in people who have arthritis. Taking minerals in a solution and consuming a diet that includes grains and legumes is recommended. Vitamin C is essential to supplement because it reduces inflammation and helps synovial fluid lubrication so joints can move with a better range of motion. Foods that contain Vitamin C are papaya, guava, broccoli, cantaloupe, strawberries, parsley, and kale. You can add a little brewers yeast to your diet to help the bones and tissues of the body. Foods to avoid when arthritis is present are dairy foods that are saturated in fat, too much meat protein, and anything with a high amount of phosphorous, like soft drinks. Pineapples have an enzyme, bromelain that is good for reducing inflammation. Cherries, cherry juice, and black currants have bioflavonoids and Vitamin C that help with the reduction of inflammation.

Having an injury or overdoing an exercise can cause harm to the muscle proteins. Pain and muscle tenderness can be symptoms of muscle damage. Almost every vitamin and mineral is utilized in the contraction, relaxation, and repair of a muscle. Vitamin C plus bioflavonoids and Vitamin E can reduce muscle soreness and increase healing time. Aloe Vera juice is an anti-inflammatory and helps to dilate capillaries and increase blood supply to the injured area. Also, pineapple, ginger, and turmeric help to reduce inflammation and can stimulate circulation.

When you have tendonitis, it is essential that you do everything it takes to nourish the body so the tendon heals entirely. The body depends on good blood supply to heal the tissues, especially the tendons. Magnesium combined with calcium is good for your bones and it is also good for tendons and other tissues. You need the tendon to repair with the least amount of scar tissue possible. Supplementation can help heal an injury quicker with less scar tissue. Bioflavonoids and Vitamin C are great to add to your diet. Zinc and B complex vitamins are helpful to speed the healing process and reduce inflammation.

Nutrition can assist with the symptoms of carpal tunnel syndrome. The tunnel of the wrist is very small for all the structures to pass through, so any compression or swelling in that area can cause numbness and tingling in the hand. B complex vitamins can reduce inflammation and symptoms of carpal tunnel. 250 milligrams of magnesium and one tablespoon of borage or flax seed oil can help muscles and ligaments to loosen up and function better. Vitamin C and bioflavonoids aid in healing ligaments and assist with decreasing inflammation.

It is in your best interest to eat a balanced and nutritious diet to stay healthy. In your job, you are exposed to a lot of germs due to the close contact with your client. It is very important to live a healthy lifestyle and eliminate the factors that weaken the body's immune system. In conjunction with proper nutrition, you also need to supplement your body with good bacteria in the form of probiotics. Pay attention to what you consume and eliminate anything that is toxic to your body. Cleanse your body once every couple of months with an herbal cleanse or a detoxification fast. Bodyworkers need to remember the importance of a balanced and healthy lifestyle to support and strengthen the immune system.

Nutrition is essential for you as a bodyworker and as an athlete. I would sit in the break room at the spa and observe many therapists eating food out of the vending machines. Large amounts of chips and sodas were being consumed, instead of eating a healthy snack or meal. Fueling your body with adequate nutrition is one of the best decisions you can make for the health of your body and for the maintenance of your energy level.

General guidelines for eating healthy are:

- Balance the food you eat with physical activity.
- Eat a nutritionally adequate diet from a variety of foods.
- Eat a diet low in saturated fat and low in cholesterol.
- Pick a diet with whole grains, fruits, vegetables, and legumes.
- Choose a diet that is low or moderate in sugar.
- Prepare foods with a small amount of salt, if any.
- Drink alcohol in moderation.
- Eat protein in moderate amounts and mostly from plant sources.
- Try to avoid food additives and processed foods as much as possible.

Chapter Eighteen

Energizing Your Chakras with Food

As a bodyworker, you have to think about nutrition in a new way. What you eat affects your life because there is a cause and effect that happens in your body from your diet and your lifestyle choices. You need three basic substances to support your life processes. These substances are food, air, and water. Air and water were automatic in the past when there was not any pollution, but have to be taken into consideration these days. Food consumes a lot of time since we have to gather it, prepare it, eat it, and digest it. You should come to some type of understanding when it comes to your relationship with food. For some people their relationship with food is not a conscious connection and it should be.

Eating food in an appropriate fashion means utilizing energy from nature in a peaceful way. Oxygen is brought into the body from the food you eat. When oxygen enters the body, oxygen energy shifts into the lungs. The lungs are connected to the heart chakra and the extra oxygen that enters the body helps to equalize the energy between the upper and lower chakras. Oxygen stress or depletion can happen in the body from eating a poor diet. It is important to eat foods high in oxygen to avoid degenerative diseases that are generally a result of hypoxia to the tissue. It is to your advantage to eat foods with high water content since water is 85 percent oxygen. Carbohydrates contain 50 percent oxygen to weight, proteins 25 percent, and fat 12 percent.

Chakras are associated with your mental, emotional, and physical activities and revitalize your body's physical energy. Each individual has seven major chakra centers that start at the base of the spine and end at the top of your head. The chakras are openings within the human body that allow life force energy to flow in and out of the aura. Each chakra is an energy center of the body and you must maintain balance between these centers for energy exchange to take place and for optimal health to occur. Two major components are needed to balance the chakras. These components are water and food and give the required energy that the physical body requires.

Chakras are affected by the kind of food you consume. Various foods can assist in the balancing, grounding, and re-energizing of each chakra. It is extremely important to have healthy eating habits so that the chakras remain balanced. Your diet should be an important part of your lifestyle because many illnesses result from poor food choices. Nutrition is a key component for keeping the chakras balanced. All food that is consumed has certain vibrational qualities that correlate to each chakra. It is necessary to nourish your body and fuel your chakras with proper nutrition. Take a look at the food listed under each chakra to help you be mindful about your food choices. You can help bring balance to your chakras through eating a balanced and nutritious diet.

The root chakra is the first chakra and is found at the base of the spine. It is known as muladhara and it means foundation. This chakra is associated with the earth element. The root chakra is connected to the feet chakras and they are connected to the vibratory frequencies of the earth. Chakra one is balanced with foods that are physically oriented. Starting your day by eating breakfast is one way to take care of your body. A diet that includes protein is important because it connects us to the earth and grounds us. As you begin your day, start with grounding foods and then allow your energy to travel up through the chakras.

Root vegetables such as carrots, potatoes, parsnips, radishes, beets, onions, and garlic are helpful for grounding yourself. Rhubarb is very good for rising energy from the root through the spine. Protein rich foods like eggs, beans, tofu, and peanut butter are excellent sources to fuel the root chakra. You should include spices to feed this chakra. Some examples of spices you can add to your food are horseradish, paprika, chives, cayenne, and black pepper.

To make a juice to energize this chakra, juice:

Three stalks of rhubarb (do not eat the leaves because they are toxic)
Two apples
One orange
Drink and enjoy!

This drink helps to balance right and left-brain activity. If you are feeling spaced out, disconnected or separated from your body, try these food examples listed above to balance the root chakra. As you eat or drink these foods, think to yourself, I am deeply connected and rooted to the earth.

The sacral chakra is the second chakra and is the focal point of emotion, creativity, and sexual consciousness. It is known as swadhista and is associated with the water element. Emotions have a strong effect on this chakra. For this reason, emotions need to be felt and confirmed. Through this chakra, you will learn to respect your own boundaries and reconnect with yourself. Practicing integrity is the key to keeping this chakra balanced.

Sweet fruits can help to balance this water element chakra. Melons, mangoes, strawberries, passion fruit, oranges and coconut would be very beneficial for the sacral chakra. Include honey, almonds and walnuts in your diet and add the spices of cardamon, vanilla, carob, cinnamon and caraway seeds to balance the sacral chakra.

A drink you can make to balance the sacral chakra is to juice:

One mango
Four tangerines
Six strawberries
Drink this juice thirty minutes before any breakfast foods.

To prepare this second chakra drink you will blend:

Two cut up peaches
One cup almond milk or yogurt
One teaspoon chopped mint leaves
One cup grated ginger
One tablespoon of sweetener (agave and honey are good alternatives)
Two tablespoons of ground pumpkin seeds or one tablespoon of flax seed oil

This drink will heal your body and wake up your senses. Peaches are symbolic of sensuality and contain the color of the second chakra.

If you are feeling overemotional, emotionally blocked, or unbalanced sexually use these ideas to balance the sacral chakra. Think to yourself, I feel and validate my emotions and sexuality as a natural expression on this earth. I permit any imbalances to release so I can express myself fully.

The solar plexus chakra is called manipura and it means city of jewels. This chakra is associated with the fire element, is the third chakra, and is the seat of your personal power. It is your center of energy. In order to energize the body and balance this physical chakra you need a good diet, plenty of rest, and exercise. This chakra is balanced with whole grains. It is best to avoid refined starches and simple sugars for the health of this chakra.

Granola and grains help to balance the solar plexus chakra. Whole grain pasta, bread, rice, flax seeds, and sunflower seeds are good choices of grains. Dairy foods such as milk, cheese and yogurt are beneficial as well. Valuable spices for this chakra are ginger, mint, fennel, turmeric, and cumin.

To balance and energize the solar plexus center you will blend:

One banana
One fourth a cup of coconut, soy, or almond milk
A dash of cinnamon
Drink and enjoy!

Papaya is known as the universal healer in Indonesia. The papaya includes the enzyme papain and is good for digestion. Pineapple also contains an enzyme called bromelain that helps to suppress the appetite and reduce inflammation.

To energize the solar plexus chakra, blend:

One cup of cut pineapple
One papaya, cut into pieces
One cup of apple juice or purified water
One teaspoon of dried peppermint leaves
Serve and feel the benefits from this digestive tonic.

Are you feeling egoless or egotistical? Are you procrastinating any important goals? If so, this chakra may need to be balanced. When eating or drinking to stabilize the sacral chakra, think to yourself, I take appropriate action on my own path. I allow my intuition to lead me and allow myself to rest and take action when it is appropriate.

The heart chakra is the fourth chakra and is known as anahata. This chakra is associated with the air element. The quality of air we breathe and the depth of how we breathe is connected to love. The balance of how you love yourself and how you love others is essential to having a healthy heart chakra. The love of others must come from a strong sense and love of the self. The thymus gland is associated with this chakra and is important for your immunity. Many vegetables help to create balance in the heart chakra because they are the product of the vital energy of the sun. Vegetables are the product of natural earth processes provided in a state of natural balance.

Leafy greens such as spinach, kale, and dandelion greens are beneficial for the heart chakra. Air vegetables are important for your immunity and include vegetables such as broccoli, cauliflower, cabbage, and celery. Green tea is a good liquid to drink and basil, sage, thyme, cilantro, and parsley are excellent herbs to include for this center. The color green is the vibratory color of this chakra. Kiwis are green and are a great example of a fruit for the heart chakra. Kiwis contain a high percentage of Vitamin C and contain antioxidants that neutralize free radicals.

To keep the heart chakra balanced:

Cut and peel three kiwis
Include a half a cup of raspberries
A half a cup of pink grapefruit juice
One teaspoon of spirulina
Blend on high for one to two minutes
Drink and think about boosting your immunity as you open your heart center.

Are you feeling judgmental toward yourself or other people? Do you feel like you could have more compassion? As you consume this drink, think to yourself, my love and compassion for myself allows me to feel for others. I allow myself to breathe in love and peace.

The throat chakra is the fifth chakra and is known as vissudha. It means purification and is represented by the color blue. This chakra is the seat of expression. Your expression can manifest in many creative ways. The throat chakra is associated with speaking your truth and has to do with the quality of your listening skills. Ether is the element and the thyroid is the gland that is linked to the throat chakra. Fruits are helpful for balance of the throat chakra. Fruit energy is rapidly absorbed and allows energy to travel to the upper chakras.

The shape of the thyroid is much like a butterfly. The thyroid thrives on iodine and mineral rich food and drinks. Vegetables that are grown in iodine-rich soil are beneficial for the thyroid. Otherwise, sea vegetables are a great source of an iodine rich source. You will want to avoid iodine rich foods if you are allergic to iodine or shellfish. Coconut milk helps to balance the thyroid and parathyroid and contain essential fatty acids that are necessary for your body.

Ginger is a good food for your throat and for communication. Also, tart or tangy fruits such as lemon, lime, and grapefruit are excellent for the throat chakra. Tree grown fruits such as apples, pears, and plums are good to energize this chakra. To balance the throat chakra, drink plenty of water, fruit juice, tea, and add lemon grass to your diet.

To balance your communication, juice:

Two medium apples
Two kale leaves
Two collard green leaves

A cube of ginger
Chill, drink, and enjoy!

To help balance your communication needs, combine:

One cup of coconut water or juice
A half of a cup of blueberries
A half of a cup of almond or soymilk
One tablespoon of flax seed oil
Blend on high and serve chilled.

Are you having trouble speaking your truth or avoiding the expression of important issues? Do you talk more than you listen? Do you speak the truth with value in your communication? Think to yourself, I speak my truth with value and without fear. I listen and express my opinion when appropriate.

The third eye or brow chakra is the seat of vision and imagination. The third eye chakra is known as ajna, is associated with light, and is related to the pituitary gland. Visual imagery is associated with this chakra. Creativity starts with a vision. This center is where you can use clairvoyance, which will give you the ability to see the truth.

When you practice silence daily, you develop your intuition. As you build your intuition, you will learn to let the ego drop away and allow the intuition of the third eye chakra to proceed with truth. If you try to satisfy your needs from your ego, the third eye will remain closed. When you let the lower chakras work from intuition, you will come from a place of deeper security. Keep in mind that the body will act out from fear, stress, and anger. When the intuition is not used, emotions can be repressed, especially when you are attached to a specific expectation.

Any indigo or purple foods will serve this chakra. Some good examples of these foods are red grapes, blackberries, and raspberries. Blueberries are considered a superfood that contains antioxidants and phytonutrients and are considered very valuable for the throat chakra. Liquids such as red wine and grape juice help to balance and open this chakra. Lavender and poppy seeds are also very beneficial for this center and mangoes are full of bioflavonoids, fiber, potassium, and vitamin C.

To maintain a balanced third eye chakra, combine:

One cup of blackberries
A mango (pitted and chopped)
One half cup of purified water
One tablespoon of flaxseed oil
Blend and serve chilled.

To energize and awaken the throat chakra, combine:

The juice of five lemons
Four cups of watermelon chunks
One cup of pomegranate juice
Two tablespoons of agave nectar
Blend on high for one minute and drink.

The crown chakra is the seventh chakra and is seen as a thousand-petal lotus at the top of the head. The seventh chakra is known as sahasrara. Fasting and detoxification will help to fuel this chakra. Frankincense, sage, and myrrh can be used to smudge your aura and the environment around you.

Your thoughts come from this chakra. If you meditate and learn to control your thoughts, you will realize the power that your thoughts have on your body and your life. Your thoughts create your life, as your reality. The crown chakra acts as a gateway from the universe and is an entry and exit point for the physical body. Your higher self is connected through the crown chakra.

Before meditating, drink lemon barley tea by combining:

A half of a cup of pearl barley
Four cups of water
Simmer for 20-25 minutes
Add the juice of a lemon and one teaspoon of agave or honey
This drink can be consumed hot or cold and is a great cleanser for the kidneys

If you want to meditate or connect when doing healing work, blend:

One pint of blackberries
Two cups of purified water
One tablespoon of honey or agave nectar
The juice of one orange
Serve this sweet and light drink chilled to help you connect to your higher self.

All of the chakra energy centers need to be kept in balance. In addition to the major energy centers there are also hand and feet chakras that are minor energy centers that receive and disperse energy. The hand and feet chakras need to be kept open and cleared as you do your work. The hand chakras are located in the palm and are smaller than the main chakras along the spine. The hands are mostly connected to the heart chakra and have minor connections to the throat and brow chakras. Your hands filter and release healing energy. A person that uses their hands extensively will benefit from lemon verbena tea or lemonade made from juiced lemons. This tea is especially important for computer users because it clears away some of the absorption of the electromagnetic energy.

The feet chakras are located in the arch of the foot and are connected to the root chakra. The feet chakras help you to ground and connect to the earth energy. To stimulate each foot chakra, try to walk without your shoes in the dirt or grass daily to feel your connection to the earth and stay grounded.

Earth-grown fruits and vegetables assist in the opening and clearing of each foot chakra. Potatoes, carrots, and apples are good examples of earth-grown fruits and vegetables.

Eat from a wide range of colors and remember that each color contains a vibration and the energetic frequency it holds will help to balance your body and your chakras. These drinks are literally liquid conductors of your thoughts. When you focus positive thoughts and intentions onto your food or drink, you have the ability to affect different parts of your body.

To energize your chakras:

- Eat live food.
- Consume a balanced and nutritious diet.
- Eat whole grains.
- Maintain a diet that contains many colors.
- Balance each chakra.
- Be conscious of your food choices.
- Understand what your body needs at specific times.

Chapter Nineteen

Protection for Body, Mind, and Spirit

Everything you do takes energy. The energy of molecules moving in and around you can take place in many different ways. Energy can be expressed as effort or it can be expressed for basics of living like breathing, digestion, or thinking. You spend a particular amount of energy on certain things in your life. If you spend little or no time or energy on something, you are not giving it much energy. If you spend a lot of time and energy on something, you are giving energy to it. You can give energy positively like doing something kind for yourself or others. You can also give energy negatively like worrying or not being nice to someone. It actually takes more effort to give your energy in a negative way than it does to give it in a positive way.

It is necessary for you to be aware of the energy in and around you because whether you realize it or not, energy is all around you. Everything in this world is vibrating at different rates and giving off energy. An exchange of energy occurs when two people interact. You have to be aware of all energy exchanges when doing bodywork because whether you know it or not, you are running energy when you do bodywork.

The energy field is made up of the aura and the chakras. The aura surrounds the human body and is composed mostly of electromagnetic radiation. The aura has seven layers and extends up to four feet from the human body. Each layer represents a different part of your energy and exudes a different color. The aura constantly changes and is affected by your thoughts, intentions, creativity, and emotions.

The human aura has regions of the body that serve as energy warehouses. These depots store energy and transmit that energy to your organs and meridians. The aura is the result of the energy field. This force field is made up of an energy rising up through the body and another energy moving downward. These two energies cross when moving through the body. Main energy centers are located where these energies cross.

Your body contains seven basic energy centers that are located in the energy body from the top of the head to the lower torso. (19.1) These energy centers connect to major nerve ganglia and are called chakras. Chakras are transmitters of energy and are like a whirling vortex. This vortex can be sucked in or pushed out if it is out of balance. A chakra that is spinning at a rate that is too fast or too slow is not in balance. A balanced chakra is at a level of harmony when it spins at a rate relative to the others and takes only the energy it needs. Chakras reflect the physical, mental and spiritual parts of a person. When negative emotions are stuck in the energy field, a chakra can become dysfunctional. Physical injuries and moral issues can also create imbalances in the chakras and can result in disease.

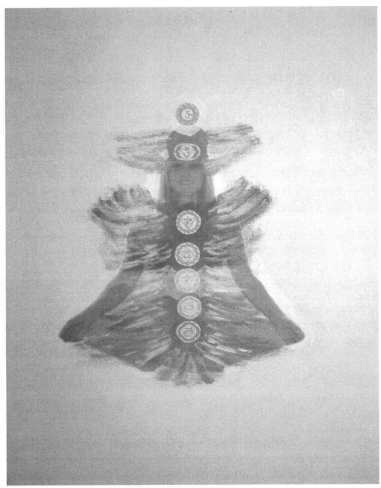

19.1 The Chakras

Think of your chakras like a computer. The chakras store the programming of your life and how you function. The first chakra, located under the belly button in the lower torso, is like your survival file. The first chakra contains what you eat, exercise habits, how you anger and where you live. It holds your tribal beliefs. The second chakra provides the nurturing and sexuality files. This chakra holds your views of respect, ethics, and preferences. The third chakra is the program of power and is the site of personal will. These three chakras are all physical in nature. The fourth chakra is associated with unconditional love and heart felt issues. The fifth chakra deals with communication. In other words, how you speak your truth and listen to what others have to say. These two chakras are emotional in nature and are the gateway to spiritual growth. The sixth chakra is the third eye where intuition lies and the seventh chakra is your connection to source and spirituality. The upper chakras deal with perception and intellect and are like motherboards of a computer. People are internal computers of different models. Each of us is unique and programmed with a specific language. Everyone uses his or her own distinct operating systems.

Good health occurs when your energy field is strong and the energy in your aura is moving freely. Your energy field or aura is healthy when it is balanced and when the protective layer is elastic and flexible like rubber. If you keep your energy balanced and flowing, the aura will remain strong and run at a high vibrational level. If you do not know how to protect your energy field, it can be running at a low vibrational level and your protective layer can become vulnerable and porous. When your energy is running at a low vibrational level, it can leave your aura vulnerable. You can help protect your energy field with many different tools. Protecting your own energy field and learning how to conserve your energy are important aspects when you are holding a therapeutic and healing environment.

The toolbox for protecting your vital energy includes: centering, grounding, decording, cleansing, and shielding. Centering is very important for being present in the here and now. Being present is crucial for healing energy to continue flowing. Your core is the center of gravity. Your center is also the point that leads your intuition and helps the whole body move more gracefully and effortlessly. To locate your center, place your palms on your belly. Create a triangle with the thumbs touching above the belly button and the fingers touching below the belly button. You can also put one had under the belly button and one hand directly opposite on the back while breathing into this area. If you notice yourself feeling off balance, take a moment to breathe into this area and bring yourself back to the center.

Connect with the earth's energies by grounding your feet into the earth via roots or tubes. Ground your energy down into the earth and draw the earth's energy up. Another way to ground yourself is to stand with both feet flat on the ground and visualize a cord dropping from above you and down through your crown chakra. Feel the other end of the cord connecting down through your feet and into mother earth. Let white light from the upper cord travel from the top of your head through your feet. Inhale and breathe green light up from mother earth all the way up through your crown chakra. Exhale. Inhale and breathe violet from the crown down through the feet. Exhale and feel the feet contacting the ground. When you feel completely grounded, slowly open your eyes and feel yourself in the present moment.

During a session, some of your vital energy is transferred into the client's body and some of their energy is conducted into you through contact. "Cording" is described as a line of life force that runs through two people. It is through this cord that energy is exchanged. Most cording happens on the unconscious level. Therefore, you must know that you have the ability to use certain techniques to protect yourself against any unwanted energy. The secret to protecting yourself is to be aware of energy flowing in and out of you. Always decord or cut the healing cord when ending a session. Decording is unplugging or cutting off any energy cords that have formed during a session. Hold the client's feet and visualize the cord being cut with scissors. Seal both ends of the cord with white or green light.

Cleansing your energy can be done with a simple brush of the aura or it can be done with thought. To brush the aura, place your hands in front of your body with the palms facing in. Sweep your hands around your body and smooth out your aura just like you would pet a dog. Cleanse your energy using images of white light, water, or fire to remove blocks and clear debris from your aura. Visualize shields around your aura to deflect and neutralize any unwanted energy. You can also wash your hands up to the elbows in cold water to stop the energy flow. While washing your hands, think to yourself, may all negative thoughts, feelings, and emotions be washed down the drain at this time. Thank you.

Before you do any type of bodywork, it is a good idea to cement your aura. Visualize your aura around you. As the aura expands outward, band and cement it with the colors of white, gold, and violet. See white light and energy entering into your crown and flowing through your hands. Think to yourself, let my aura be surrounded with white, violet, and gold light. Allow only positive energy and love to enter and exit my aura.

You can place columns of light around you to dispel negativity. Visualize silver or platinum columns surrounding you or another person to neutralize any negative energy. Gold and white light help to surround and protect your energy. You can also put these columns around your massage room to protect each session.

You can utilize crystals to assist in the protection of your energy. Crystals can help to absorb and protect your aura and are efficient in cleansing the aura and transmuting negative energy. Crystals carry particular vibrational rates and work through energy resonance and vibration. When you place a crystal in your aura, the vibrational rate can change within your aura. Quartz crystal has many modern uses. Quartz has piezoelectric properties that conduct electricity and can produce sound waves. Quartz is also used as a laser in the medical field and in computer chips in the technology field. Your body contains a measured electrical vibration and crystals can be used to bring balance to the chakras and the aura. Some crystals are calm and sedative, whereas other crystals can help to energize or activate an area or the entire body. Crystals regulate the body's vibrational quality and bring balance to your energy system.

Crystals must be cared for before you use them. Once you have selected a stone, you must clear it. You can clear a crystal by placing it under running water, in sea salt, or under the light of a full moon. Crystals such as selenite can be damaged by water so sea salt or moonlight would be a better option. On the other hand, citrine, kyanite, and azeztukite contain properties that are self-clearing and never need to be cleared. Crystals can be worn as a necklace, ring, or bracelet. You can also carry a crystal in a pouch and put it in your pocket to keep near your body. You will want to consult a good reference source for specifics on crystal care, properties, and cleansing. When you receive a new crystal, hold it in your hands and have the intention of using the crystal for only light and love.

Many crystals help to shield the aura and align the chakras. You can utilize crystals for this and many other reasons. You can program a crystal if you want to receive certain qualities from it. Be precise when programming the crystal and use intent. Hold it in your hand and think of a specific phrase as you repeat it 20 times. Take a few deep breaths and seal the energy in with white light surrounding you and the crystal. Crystals need to be cared for. They need to be protected from chipping or breaking and they need to be cleared and re-programmed often. The one thing to keep in mind is the fact that you are working with many people's energies throughout the day. It is always a good idea to regularly cleanse the crystals you are wearing after a day of working.

Clear quartz has many uses. Clear quartz is a very powerful healer and energy amplifier. It absorbs, releases, stores, and regulates energy. It also shields the aura. Smokey quartz will help you to ground your energy, while absorbing electromagnetic radiation, and neutralizing negative energy. It is very good at reducing pain but smokey quartz needs to be cleared often. Citrine is energizing and dissipates negative energy. Citrine helps to cleanse the chakras, especially the solar plexus and the sacral chakra. This stone also helps with abundance if you place a piece in your wallet and hold the intention of prosperity. Hematite is an excellent stone for grounding and protecting your energy. It prevents negative energy from entering your aura. Kunzite has a high vibrational quality and is a protective stone that transmutes negativity. Kunzite forms a protective shield around your aura when worn.

Stones such as labadorite deflect negative energy from the aura and keep the energy in the aura while during your healing work. Labadorite is known as a "healer's stone" because it works from a spiritual level and helps you to trust in yourself and the universe. Obsidian is a dark stone that forms a protective shield around the aura and forms a cord from the root chakra into the earth. Obsidian absorbs negative energy and needs to be cleared often. Black tourmaline protects against electromagnetic radiation and connects with the base chakra. It helps with grounding earth energy while increasing physical vitality. Blue tourmaline is a wonderful stone for a healer because it prevents negative energy from staying in the aura. It also carries the energy of peace and balances the throat chakra. Turquoise is a great stone because it provides the wearer with protection. It is also a purification stone and dispels negative energy especially in the case of a physical injury. Turquoise helps to strengthen the meridians and energy field of the body. Rose quartz purifies the heart and keeps the energy flow open from the heart through the hands. Rose quartz helps you to love yourself and, in turn, love others. Amethyst is a protective stone with a high vibration. It transmutes any negative energy into love. Amethyst heightens your intuition and brings out each person's psychic gifts. Charoite is a great stone for healer since it aids in transformation and dispels fear. Charoite encourages change to a higher vibration and helps to cleanse the aura. This stone also forms a connection from the heart and crown chakra and helps you to walk your spiritual path with awareness.

When using these crystals to help balance your chakras place a stone on a certain part of the body and leave it on for 15 minutes. Relax and breathe thinking only positive thoughts. You can place a stone on a specific chakra or you can position one stone on each chakra. Also, crystals or stones can be placed above the head and below the feet, depending on the results you want to achieve.

Affirmations are useful for developing a positive mindset. Affirmations are positive statements for particular situations and are repeated over and over to make an impact on the subconscious mind. Affirmations are very helpful to imprint positive thoughts in your mind and discard negative thoughts. The effectiveness of an affirmation has to do with repetition, intention, and desire. Many times a person will repeat a negative thought concerning a specific situation and can attract negative situations into their life. Affirmations program the mind just like you would program a computer. The repeated words help you to focus your mind and transform behaviors, thought patterns, mental reactions, and habits. The key to success is to repeat each affirmation and keep the statement short so you can remember it. Choose only positive words and experience the feeling you will have once you achieve the outcome. Always affirm in the present tense and see each outcome transform as you attract what you truly want in your life.

Some affirmations you can use:

> I have abundant energy.
> I am safe and protected at all times.
> I am happy and healthy everyday and everyway.
> My body is healthy and functioning optimally.
> I radiate love and happiness.
> I am surrounded by love.
> Everything is getting better and better everyday.
> I am successful in everything I do.

The more you protect your energy and the more psychically strong you are, the less likely your energy will be drained or taken away. Heal yourself first and then you will have more strength to heal others. Remember that like attracts like. If some type of energy or thought form resonates between you and your client, you can sympathize in some way. The universal law of attraction states that if something is alike energetically, it is attracted magnetically. A major reason to protect your energy is because you can sympathize and feel on certain levels that is not your energy. It is essential to be empathetic instead of sympathetic and recognize any energy or feeling that is not yours.

Remember that an energy cord is formed between you and your client when a healing session begins. Decording from the client at the conclusion of the session and clearing your energies between sessions is imperative to your well-being. Always see yourself cut the cord with scissors at the conclusion of the session. See yourself transmitting energy to them but know that you do not have to take on their energy. Realize that you need to have awareness and be able to control how much energy is being transferred. You can allow for a certain amount of energy per client but you cannot give all of yourself to each and every client. Only give what is needed for each client and conserve enough energy for yourself at the end of the day.

As mentioned previously, grounding should always be a priority before each session. If you start a healing session ungrounded, you will have inadequate energy to help the person in need and your energy will become drained quickly. Starting a session with deficient energy creates an environment for negative emotions to develop. Depletion of your own health can start to occur, if you are practicing without grounding yourself over a long period of time.

The earth is full of energy and you must be come skilled at accessing this energy. The earth has abundant energy for you to make use of so take what you need and use it in a positive way. The earth is the base for which all life exists. You are privileged to connect with the energy of nature and improve other people's lives. It is essential for you to improve your own energy by interacting with the source of energy outdoors, in nature.

Lying or sitting on the earth is excellent to clear your energy and build an energy reserve to do your healing work. When utilizing the energy of nature, your first step is to pay attention to the energy of the earth. Lie with your back on the ground. Bring awareness to your spine as it contacts the earth. Release each section of the spine against the earth. Relax the muscles and let the whole body melt into the ground. Bring your attention further down into the earth. Allow your body to release waste energy into the earth. Bring your attention to specific parts of your body that have pain and visualize the earth bringing healing energy to that place. Stay in this position for 10-20 minutes, depending on the rate your energy releases.

The second approach to accessing earth energy is to stand while contacting the earth's energy through the feet. Start doing this exercise for just for a minute or two at a time to feel the sensation through the feet. Pay close attention to your body and if you loose concentration just wiggle your toes. Developing your connection with the earth is done with concentration and practice. Repeat this exercise each day as you practice with different variations. Open and soften your feet while feeling a sensation of your feet sinking into the earth and visualize your feet entering the ground. Concentrate only on the sensations of the feet.

In a few weeks, try some more difficult variations. Stand barefoot and in silence while you visualize beams of light moving through the soles of the feet and into the earth. This exercise is very empowering and important because your body will become more easily filled with the energy of the earth. As time goes by, start feeling the sensations in the feet and then move your attention up into the legs and upper body. When practicing these exercises, notice any feelings of tingling, warmth, calmness, relaxation, and subtle vibration as the energy is exchanged.

The standing exercise should be done everyday. Standing is how most of your work is done and it is essential that you learn how to access this energy. This exercise should be performed either in the morning or at night. Perform the exercise as needed when your body is feeling depleted. Never attempt to do a bodywork session without first filling up your body's energy through the feet. To do a session without admitting the earth's energy and filling up your energy can deplete your own energy reserve. Doing bodywork without grounding yourself, on a frequent basis, could result in disease of your body. These exercises can be done indoors if no other options are available. If doing your work indoors and you need to access more energy, just visualize your feet on the ground and see the energy being pulled up through the feet.

The feet are the interface with the earth. Energy flows through the organs and chakras and end in the feet. Go barefoot outdoors as much as you can and cleanse the waste energy from your feet each day by standing on the earth. Protect your energy by utilizing these tools every day, especially on the days that you work. Build an energy reserve so you have abundant energy to perform at your highest potential.

Chakra Meditation

Visualize a beautiful rainbow above your head filled with every color of the rainbow.

Pull the color red down through the body. Allow the body to be bathed in red, giving strength and resilience to every cell.

Bring the color orange down from the rainbow and let this beautiful color fill the whole body.

Next, see the color yellow moving down into the solar plexus and feel the body warm up with the color of the sun.

Allow the color green to move through your heart area. Feel the healing power of green embrace your body fully.

Visualize the color blue bathing the throat area. See blue cleansing and rejuvenating this area.

Fill your body with purple. Release this purple color between your eyes. Allow this color to cleanse the body of pain and stress.

See white light entering through the crown of the head and enveloping the entire body. Feel white light cleanse each part of you while it bathes each and every cell.

Breathe slowly and deeply seeing any darkness in your body dissipate. When you are ready, slowly open your eyes and come back to the present moment.

Feel yourself completely relaxed and renewed.

This exercise will generally take five minutes but it can last as long as you would like it to. Experience the difference in your body before the mediation versus after.

Many tools can be utilized to balance and protect your energy. You can use visualization, yoga postures, and breathing to balance your chakras and protect your energy body. Daily meditation can clear the mind, ground you, and relax your physical body. Meditation also helps to keep the chakras and aura clear, aligned, and balanced. It is essential for you to keep your energy level at a high vibrational rate and keep yourself protected while maintaining a therapeutic presence.

Ways you can protect your body, mind, and spirit:

- Meditation
- Visualization
- Positive Affirmations
- Yoga postures
- Breathing
- Decording
- Shielding
- Cleansing
- Centering
- Grounding
- Crystals
- Utilize nature's energy

Notes

Chapter Twenty

Self-Care For the Bodyworker

Your career will be more fulfilling when the physical, psychological, social, and spiritual aspects of your life are balanced. Being healthy means that all of these various facets are working together harmoniously. When body, mind, and spirit are all incorporated a higher level of wellness can be achieved. The success or lack of success of a career in bodywork is dependent on how you expend your energy, how you care for yourself, how you learn to receive and give back to yourself. Burnout in this career is very likely if self-care is not being practiced. You must discover a way to find balance in your life. Balance happens when different parts of your life are in proportion to each other. The relationship you have with yourself is the basis for all energy exchanges. If you distinguish what your needs and wants are and attend to your own needs first, you will feel more free and empowered. Making time in your life to practice meditation, breathing, and yoga will help you give back to yourself and will offer you the time needed for self-reflection.

Make an effort to balance your physical self first. The physical part of your job can cause wear and tear on your body and lead to burnout. Important components when caring for your physical body would include: exercise, nutrition, proper body mechanics, and plenty of rest. You must use your body in a wise manner when doing massage. Using your body incorrectly can lead to excessive muscle tension in the upper trapezius, erector spinae, wrist extensors, and finger flexors. An asymmetric stance such as warrior pose is the best to use in a lot of cases. When applying pressure, try to keep the joints stacked to conserve your energy and lessen muscle overuse and misuse. Keep your body as relaxed as possible and stay behind each stroke while leaning into the tissue beneath you. These few concepts will also feel better to your client while you are performing each technique. Increase the amount of massages you do gradually and take adequate breaks in between sessions. The key to longevity in this career is good body mechanics and proper self-care.

Another key factor when striving for longevity in this career is to get the proper amount of physical activity in addition to the work you are doing. Exercise increases circulation and delivers oxygen to the cells. Exercise builds strength in your body gradually and ensures you the endurance you need to perform your job. It is very important to warm up, lengthen, and stretch the soft tissues before exercising. Make sure you use good body mechanics when working out to avoid injury. Exercise is highly beneficial for bodyworkers to increase energy, maintain stamina, and reduce injury. Start building strength early in your career, particularly while you are still in school. You can start by walking and doing lunges to build strength in your legs. Begin building up the strength slowly in your arms because these small muscles have a lot of repetitive motions to do and need endurance to perform these motions.

Psychological self-care is essential for you as a bodyworker. Anytime you share personal space with a client, grounding and centering become very important. Grounding creates a barrier space between you and your client and centering helps you to stay focused with your client in the moment. When grounding yourself prior to a session, remind yourself that you are only a facilitator of the healing energy being transferred to your client. With this thought in mind, you will remain humble and empower your client to be responsible for their own health and healing. Mental centering clears the mind and helps you to keep your focus on the client and their needs. Using rhythmic breathing is one of the best examples for focusing on the present moment and will help your mind to stay focused and keep it from wandering.

Education and having fun are other ways of taking care of yourself and deterring burnout. Education stimulates the mind and learning helps to keep you up-to-date on the latest information. Reading, writing, and taking continuing education classes are essential. Broadening your knowledge base will not only make you a better therapist but it will create more enthusiasm in your career and make your massage better.

Healthy relationships are essential to your mental well-being. Relationships are about energy exchange. You need to learn how to balance the energy flow between you and your partners, friends, and family members. Socializing can be a great energy boost and lots of fun at the same time.

Spiritual self-care should be very important to you, no matter what religious affiliation you are. Spirituality plays a big role in your health and well-being. Having some type of spirituality in your life helps you to have faith, accept life's challenges, and helps you to move in the direction of wellness.

As a bodyworker, you can burnout physically, mentally, and emotionally. Practice self-care daily to protect your energy and longevity. Balance your work with education, play, and social activities to deter burnout. Consider taking a vacation often and do something that is nurturing for yourself. Make play dates with your friends and do things that you enjoy. Life will not be as much of a challenge if you have more fun.

Start your day with grounding and meditation via yoga, breathing, and visualization. This practice will increase the energy that is needed, recharge you, and give your body a surplus of energy to work with. If you start your day with an energy deficit you are setting yourself up for burnout, exhaustion, and injury. Think of your energy as a bank account and do not let your account overdraw and become depleted. If you build your energy up and create a reserve, you will have excess energy to draw off of.

Sleep and rest are vital for repairing and restoring the body. Make sure you get adequate rest to renew your energy for the next day. Think of your physical body as a battery and realize that you charge your battery when you rest or sleep. The body goes into repair mode when you go into deep sleep and so it is necessary to get adequate sleep to avoid injury. Sleeping at least eight hours each night is essential to charging your battery and building up your bank account.

There are many ways to get better quality sleep. It is a good idea to reduce caffeine intake at least six hours prior to going to sleep. Caffeine can keep you awake and stay in your body up to eight hours. You should definitely prohibit the use of nicotine. Nicotine is a stimulant to the central nervous system and reduces the overall amount of oxygen in the blood. Avoid alcohol because it can disturb sleep and result in less restorative sleep. Exercise can enhance your sleep but it is best done in the morning, late afternoon, or early evening. Do something relaxing before bedtime. You can meditate, stretch, or take a hot bath before retiring. Finally, create the ideal sleeping environment by keeping your bedroom dark and quiet. The setting should be comfortable with the proper temperature and sleeping support. A good mattress and pillow that gives your back and neck support are essential to a good night's rest.

A nutritious diet for the bodyworker is essential. Live foods fuel your body and give you increased energy. Preservatives can create waste products in the body and sometimes can cause pain in the joints and muscles. Eat nutritious foods that will fuel your body and avoid anything that will deplete your energy body. Caffeine, alcohol, and refined sugar are examples of substances that deplete you of your energy.

Therapists need to receive massage. This statement should be a given, but unfortunately it is not. You cannot expect to help others if you are not well physically and balanced in all areas of your life. Take some time out to get a massage and either pay for it or trade with a friend. Receiving massage is a necessary component to your self-care routine.

The benefits of receiving massage are numerous. Most importantly, massage supports your health and well-being and helps to prevent injury by keeping the tissues supple and aligned correctly. Massage improves circulation and is a key to health by removing waste products from the body. Adhesions and fibrous tissue are broken up with massage, allowing the muscles to glide smoothly alongside each other. Massage aids in flexibility and reduces injury.

Self-massage is another key to a healthy career! Massage helps to reduce muscle tension and increases blood flow to the tissues. Self-massage is a proven technique for reducing muscle tension, fatigue, and pain. You have all the tools and knowledge at your fingertips to do massage on yourself. You can utilize your own hands to help your body stay healthy. There are two advantages to massaging yourself versus getting a massage from someone else. These two reasons for self-massage are that it does not cost anything and you get immediate feedback from your body. A few ideas to receive self-massage is to massage your body in the morning when applying lotion, every time you lotion your hands you can massage tension out, and massage the stress out of your feet every night by rolling your feet over a tennis ball. You can use your own hands, a tool, or hot stones for self-massage. I also like to do a hot stone layout and lay on the stones when my back is hurting.

Make it a habit to massage your own forearms on a weekly basis. Cross-fiber friction the tendons of the forearm muscles at the medial and lateral epicondyles. Strip the flexors and extensor muscles of the forearm with cross-fiber friction and longitudinal strokes to reduce any adhesions. After you complete the self-massage, then stretch to re-align your tissues.

Work the trigger points in the upper body to relieve myofascial pain in the arms, elbows, forearms, wrists, and thumbs. Releasing trigger points can relieve pain, aching, numbness, swelling, and joint stiffness. Massage of a trigger point should be done on a daily basis and each area should be treated for 5-20 seconds. If the trigger point does not release at that time, then stop and move on to the next spot. You can work on a trigger point up to six times a day if you do not get a release the first few times. If you are not getting a release, you may not be treating the exact area. Never try to force a release to occur. Trigger points will release when you work with them on a daily basis. Your body is its own healer, so provide it with an environment that encourages healing.

Trigger points can originate in the neck, chest, upper body, and can refer pain down into the arm and hands. The pectoralis major needs to be stripped regularly and the trigger points need to be released. The pectoralis major can hold a lot of tension that is caused from the excessive pushing you perform in your work. If you have carpal tunnel syndrome or symptoms, you should deactivate the trigger points in the scalenes, serratus posterior, teres minor, pectoralis minor, triceps, coracobrachialis, brachialis, flexor carpi radialis, extensor carpi radialis brevis, supinator, pronator teres, and flexor digitorum. In the case of lateral epicondylitis, release trigger points in the extensor muscles of the forearm especially the extensor carpi radialis longus, extensor radialis brevis, and, extensor digitorum. Also include trigger point release on the supinator, triceps, infraspinatus, teres major, coracobrachialis, brachioradialis, and supraspinatus. If you have medial epicondylitis, work the trigger points in the pronators, palmarus longus, serratus anterior, triceps, latisimmus dorsi, pectoralis major, pectoralis minor and serratus posterior superior. The thumb is often a site of pain and can be given relief by releasing certain trigger points. For pain radiating into the thumb, deactivate the trigger points in the flexor carpi radialis, pronator quadratus, flexor pollicus longus, opponens pollicis, adductor pollicis, and the first dorsal interosseous between the thumb and index finger.

Trigger points can be worked with a number of different tools to save you from overworking your own hands. You can utilize the opposite forearm to strip the muscles in your other arm. If tools are not appropriate to the area, then use your hands with the least effort and strain. Use ischemic compression and hold the point up to 20 seconds until the nodule releases. You might feel a twitch in the muscle before the release occurs. You can also make a series of short, repeated strokes if the compression hurts your hands. After releasing the trigger points, always stretch the muscle to reset the resting length.

You use your energy and function much like that of a TV signal. You receive information through your physical body and just like a TV processes the information, it is only the mediator through which the energy is processed. When you interact with people, you interact with all their information. Their data is energy and you are interacting with it. This is the reason that it is important to know your own energy. When you are in tune with your energy, you can discern what is yours and make a separation with any energy that is not in alignment with your path. It is important to stay away from any mind enhancing drugs. Some people use drugs to be more sensitive and creative during a session. This approach can cause you to leave the physical body to access information and, in the process it leaves you open for negative energies to enter your aura. If you are not grounded and fully in your body, after time, your body will be full of energy that is not your own and you will not be in alignment with your highest potential. A large portion of therapists and bodyworkers are not aware of their own energy and the information that is given and received during a session. It is essential to protect your aura before, during, and after a session by utilizing centering, grounding, and visualization.

While doing a bodywork session, if you begin to feel drained, headachy, or nauseous, stop and shake out your hands. Notice how you are breathing, and if you are not breathing properly, switch to a pattern of deep and even breathing. See roots down into the earth from your feet and see white light moving through the crown to the feet. Visualize a gold shield surrounding and protecting you. Have the intent that this is universal energy, not your own, and let it flow through you.

To be a successful and efficient bodyworker you must be able to hold a strong therapeutic and healing presence with a surplus of energy. This means learning to stay grounded and present, leaving a space for healing to occur without taking on the client's pain. You must be empathetic and work within the given healing space. Most bodyworkers give their energy away because they like to help others. This leads to paying attention to other's needs before your own. Burnout can easily happen when you do not replenish yourself and put your own needs first. To maintain a healing presence, acknowledge when your energy reserves are low and find ways to nurture and fill yourself up with energy.

Developing a strong therapeutic presence is a gift to yourself and to your client. Clients will feel safe and relaxed when you are holding a healing space and when you are grounded and centered. This presence also increases your ability to feel what is going on with the client and separate the client's pain and energy from your own. This type of energetic connection guides you as you nurture and give back to yourself. Always holding a strong therapeutic presence is a great antidote for burnout.

Setting personal boundaries is another important step in protecting and taking care of yourself. Creating a boundary is healthy for you physically and energetically. Boundary setting can help you to create a better sense of self. Setting boundaries and respecting yourself is essential to any healthy relationship. The purpose of having boundaries is to take care of and protect yourself. You should learn to detach yourself from your own reactive process and stop judging yourself and others. Start setting boundaries between being and behavior.

It is imperative to learn to communicate how another person's behavior is affecting you. The formula for communicating your needs would include statements such as: I feel…, I want…, When you…. These statements help you to take responsibility for yourself and define yourself as separate. After verbalizing these statements, then you need to set the boundary. Describe the behavior that is unacceptable and then describe what action you will take to deal with the situation. You could say, "What you are doing is making me uncomfortable and if you do not stop I will have to end the session." Give the person a warning and if they do not heed the warning, then end the session. Express your feelings out loud and say what you will do if they do not stop the behavior. Do what you say you will do. Protect the boundary that you have set. It is not enough just to set boundaries; it is also important and necessary to enforce them.

You are powerless over other people's actions but you are not powerless over your own actions. You must know that you have choices. Take back your power and respect yourself and the boundaries you have set. Boundary issues may come up if you have experienced physical or sexual abuse and you have to set boundaries in order to not be a victim. If you are overextending and overworking yourself, you have to learn how and when to say no to your client. Also, pay attention to your energetic boundaries and only give as much energy as needed. Always leave enough energy for yourself.

You need to set a boundary to define your space and protect it. Boundaries can be set on the emotional, physical, mental, sexual, or spiritual levels. It is necessary to set boundaries because it is essential to caring for and defending yourself. You have to be willing to take the risk and have healthy relationships with yourself and others.

Another way to care for yourself is through the use of natural light. Get out in the sunshine on a daily basis. Sunlight enters through the eye and then travels to the pineal gland. The pineal gland produces

179

melatonin and manufactures serotonin. Serotonin helps you to sleep, keeps you calm, and decreases carbohydrate cravings. The sunlight you receive is most effective if it is unfiltered. Sunglasses, eyeglasses, and contact lenses reduce the capability of the eyes to receive the sun's rays and secrete melatonin. Also, when you wear sunglasses, the body is not able to prevent sunburn because it cannot regulate the melatonin production. Melatonin gives natural sun protection. Glass of any kind can filter out healthy rays. A moderate amount of unfiltered sunshine in the morning or late afternoon is healthy for you.

You can benefit from the contact of light through the colors of sunrises and sunsets. The colors of a sunrise will activate the upper chakras and get you ready for your day. A sunrise starts with the colors of the lower chakras and rise to the colors of the upper chakras. The colors of a sunset move in the opposite direction of a sunrise and move from the upper chakras to the lower chakras. A sunset prepares you for rest and sleep. Watching the sunrise and sunset is valuable for connecting you to nature's rhythms. Try to see the sun rise and set in an unfiltered way everyday. If it is not possible for you to be in unfiltered sunlight, at least try to get some light through a window. You will still receive benefits but unfiltered light is the most beneficial for your health.

Experiencing starlight and moonlight can also be health promoting. On the evenings prior to, during, and after a full moon, bathe in the moonlight. This will help you to recharge your energy, clear any negative energy, and manifest all of your positive intentions. Starlight can assist the opening of the mind preceding sleep and dreaming. Light is a valuable tool to help heal and assist you energetically. It is free, as well. Light added to love equals healing. When light is included in healing all possibilities are limitless.

Self-care can be very empowering. You as a bodyworker can be praised for caring for others more than yourself but this is unhealthy for you. Self-care is not selfish; it is a matter of health. It allows you to be a better spouse, friend, and therapist. Your clients will benefit more if you do take care of yourself. Clients can sense if you are depleted emotionally and may feel guilty for needing you. You serve as a role model for your clients so take care of yourself, exude positive self-confidence, and live a healthy lifestyle. Remember to receive regular massage. It is one of the most important steps in caring for yourself.

Steps to take for self-care:

- Do self-massage
- Meditate
- Take a nap
- Get a massage
- Take a vacation
- Put your own needs first
- Set healthy boundaries
- Receive unfiltered sunlight daily

Conclusion

Making use of good body mechanics is essential to the longevity of your career. The attention you pay to your body and the way you use it are very important for durability. It is essential that you pay attention to the physical, spiritual, and emotional aspects of yourself. They are all important to a healthy career. Take care of yourself physically by practicing proper breathing, yoga, connecting to the earth, and providing yourself with proper nutrition. You can diminish burnout by means of exercise, receiving massage, getting more education, and giving back to yourself. Self-care is a necessity that allows you to continue loving what you do as a profession.

The main components of good body mechanics include having awareness of your body, practicing with ease, and keeping your body moving. Other key components are observing areas of discomfort and adjusting to a more comfortable position, restoring your body, preventing injury and employing all the self-care techniques mentioned in this book. These components are the best way to keep your body in the most excellent shape. Receiving some form of touch or energy therapy is extremely important for you as a bodyworker. Feeling what is happening in your own body is of major importance. Getting some type of bodywork a couple times a month is good for your sensorimotor education. Awareness of your body should occur on a constant basis as it will help to shed light on the parts of your body that need attention. Feeling bodywork teaches you how to live in the present moment and by receiving therapy you will gain sensory awareness. If you feel the difference between muscular tension and a relaxed muscle, you can be armed with more self-awareness.

Keep your body in alignment and keep the joints stacked as you do your work. Use leverage and leaning instead of muscle strength alone to deliver each stroke. Do yoga every day to ensure the awareness of your body in alignment. Yoga keeps the joints loose and the muscles and tendons supple. Use your breath to keep your energy flowing and supply oxygen to your muscles. As you work, keep your feet on the ground to stay connected with the earth's energies. Take into account that power is transferred from the feet and to the hands to deliver the stroke. Any stroke that does not begin with the feet is using strength solely from the upper body and can lead to excessive strain and possible injury.

Injury can happen as a part of the physical occupation you perform. If injury does occur, do not be ashamed. Stand up and say something. It may help other people. Take time off to heal, nurture your body, and be gentle with yourself. Allow the injury to heal and do not resume your work until it is completely healed.

Many adjunct therapies can assist you with your work. Hydrotherapy is a great addition to prevent injury in your body and ease the pain and tension in your client's body. Heated stone therapy is very helpful for the release of tight muscles. Also, stretching and range of motion movements can be useful to release your client's tension patterns. There are many handheld tools that you can utilize to reduce strain on your hands.

Maintain an elevated energy reserve by using deep breathing, grounding, and visualization to protect your energy reserve. Protecting your own energy reserve is extremely important for your health. To keep your energy level high, you should eat nutritious foods and keep the body flexible, strong, and supple. Also, get plenty of sleep and take time to rest and revitalize to ensure that your body is repairing. It is vital to take vacations frequently and get a massage often to keep your mind clear and your body healthy.

It is important to remember that you are not the healer; you are the vehicle or mediator of the healing. You are the middle person that transfers the healing energy and the patient accepts the amount of energy the way they want to. Mediation is the transferring of energy from the source of healing energy to the patient. To be a successful mediator you have to have an open heart and clear energy flowing throughout your physical body.

Love is the energy transferred from the heart chakra, through the hands, and to the patient. You, as the mediator, need to have an open heart to do your work. Healing does not occur in the absence of love. The heart chakra works like a light switch. This light switch can be operated by focusing on certain sensations that are around the middle of the chest. The heart chakra is either open or closed to a certain extent. An open, heart chakra emanates love, health, joy and optimism. A closed heart chakra creates the energy of anger, fear, and unhappiness. Chakras are continuously expanding and contracting as they swirl around. You will know what position your heart chakra is in by how you feel. Your heart chakra is open when you feel light, happy, healthy and vibrant.

The energy of love is a miracle. Love is emitted from the heart chakra and has the capability to transform negative energy. Love is a natural energy and emotion and it can be used as an agent of change. If you work and live with an open heart, you can teach others to have an open heart.

It is important to know that light in addition to love equals healing for yourself and your clients. Pay attention to all physical (light) and emotional (love) characteristics when performing healing work. Both light and love are valuable in creating balance, health, and healing. Light healing includes stating and thinking clear intentions. Any type of energetic balancing, chakra clearing, or color therapy can help with light healing. Unfiltered sunlight or light generated by the sunrise, sunset, stars, and moonlight are effective. Also, you can wear or place crystals in your environment for assistance with light or physical healing. Love can nourish your emotional and spiritual aspects. To create healing in your life, you need to love, have faith, and release your fears. Feel grateful, pray, meditate, be kind to all living beings, and call on spiritual guidance whenever possible to assist you on your journey.

Feel the energy of love everyday. Make it a habit. Focus your attention on the center of the chest and feel this area vibrating with pink light as it emanates love. To feel more love, cleanse your energy daily by standing or lying on the earth and transform any anger by forgiving often. You must make the choice to have an open heart and to forgive someone or something when you become angry. You must intentionally choose the energy of love to maintain an open heart.

Doing healing work allows you to assist in the flow of nature's energy. You naturally conduct energy to the one in need when doing bodywork, especially when working with a positive mindset. To think that you are the healer creates arrogance and causes you to work with your ego and not your heart. It is vital that you work with humility and love instead of egotism. Do not work with your ego. Work with your heart. The moment you step into your ego and want praise or a pat on the back is the moment that your own power can be taken away, allowing your energy to become vulnerable. This is the reason you always need to stay in your body and be grounded. Allow positive healing energy to be transferred from source, through you, and then to your client.

Your thoughts create your reality. What you think is how your life will be. Think only of what you want, not of what you do not want. You would not want to manifest any of your experiences through thinking negative thoughts. Be mindful about the theory of the current of the river. The theory states that all of your desires, big or small, add to the current of the river. Everything that you have asked for is down the river. You just have to know where you can find it. Then you can have it, experience it, and live it.

Think abundance in all aspects of life. Think abundance in health, love, relationships, money, personal growth, and energy. Think of money as being fluid. Realize that a stream can symbolize your financial situation at different times in your life. In some places, the stream will move slowly and in other places it will be spilling over. Always be grateful and realize that you are supplied for today and all of your tomorrows. Just know this and trust this and it will be.

All bodyworkers have an important mission on the earth. You have the opportunity to transform people's lives. You have the power to access healthy energy, educate, and bring awareness to a large number of people through healthy touch. Take this opportunity to connect with the earth, nature, and all the people on it to bring about change and create more love.

Last, but not least, have passion for everything you do in life, especially the healing work that you do. Know that passion satisfies the spiritual need for connection. Passion makes you feel alive and gives you a feeling that you are a part of something larger than yourself. If you look around, you will see opportunities for experiencing passion everywhere. Passion powers your soul just like a battery powers a car. Your hands will put forth the passion and enthusiasm you have. If you cannot find passion, discover it by opening up your heart and letting the passion flow in.

Be strong, be healthy, and be in charge of your body and your life.

Heal yourself first, nurture yourself, and get a massage.

If you change your thoughts, you can change the environment around you.

Have the courage to dream, hope, believe, and love.

The daily practice of gratitude is the way in which abundance will come to you.

Let what you love be what you do.

Every client is a gift from the universe and has something to teach you. What do your clients bring to your life and what can you offer in their life to assist them with love and transformation?

Appendix I

Resources

I am not a physician of any kind and hereby disclaim any responsibility of any kind for groups, professionals, or tools listed here. I strongly request that you check all references for any professionals listed on this page.

Some support groups may be able to give you a reference for medical references.

Support groups:
Association for Repetitive Motion Syndromes (ARMS)
www.certifiedpst.com/arms/index.html

www.rsi-relief.com is a good site with tips on injury prevention, support, and recovery.

Sorehand e-mail discussion group and online community
www.sorehand.org/

To find a Doctor:
http://eeshop.unl.edu/findadoc.html
To find Healthcare Providers: http://eeshop.unl.edu/providers/provide2.html

Massage Table carts:
www.earthlite.com

Massage supplies and adjustable stools:
www.massagewarehouse.com

Magazine for massage therapists with the latest news and information:
www.massagemag.com

Appendix II

Self-Care Tools

The Backnobber II is s- shaped and about twenty inches long. It is portable, folds in the middle, and comes with a thirty five-page guide. The backnobber II releases trigger points in back, sides, and front.
www.pressurepositive.com

Theracane- self-massage tool shaped like a cane. Releases trigger points in hard to reach areas. Manual included.
www.theracane.com

Knobble- smooth, hard wooded tool designed like a mushroom. Fits comfortably in the hand or used for compression in different areas of the body.
www.pressurepositive.com

Yamuna Body Rolling- uses four to nine inch balls in various routines to reeducate and elongate muscles. These balls help therapists to realign tissue and release tension accumulated during a typical workday.
www.yamunabodyrolling.com

Roleo Therapeutic Massager- uses a push-pull motion between two rollers to massage the forearm muscles. Helps to reduce repetitive strain syndromes and is easy to use in your home or the office.
www.rollyourpainaway.com

Appendix III

Self-Care Tips

1. Receive massage once a week. It will keep you physically, mentally, and emotionally in touch. Massage also helps to prevent injuries and release physical and energetic toxins.
2. Set boundaries with yourself, your clients, and your family. Always make sure there is a trade of energy involved. This will prevent resentment.
3. Practice what you preach. Do what you tell your clients to do to stay healthy.
4. Make sure you are using your body correctly. Constantly monitor yourself and your actions from the inside out.
5. Take time for yourself each day to maintain your spirit. Meditate, exercise, read a book, or take a nap.
6. Do not take your job personally. You cannot fix all your clients. You are the passenger and they are the driver.
7. Take a vacation.
8. Write in a journal for physical, mental, and spiritual reasons.
9. Make your days off, your days off. Give your body time to recover.
10. Appreciate everything in your life.

Key Words

Alignment- the arrangement of the body in a straight line and relative to the position of the client's body.

Body Awareness- the ability to feel how and where you are moving your body.

Body Mechanics- the careful and efficient use of your body by incorporating leverage and alignment to reduce fatigue and prevent injury.

Bodywork- body-centered therapy that involves manipulation of the client's body as a way to maintain or improve health.

Centering- the focus of your attention and intention on the client.

Cryotherapy- the use of low temperatures in medical therapy to decrease inflammation, pain, and spasm.

Ease- lack of difficulty in doing or achieving a desired goal.

Exploration- the study or examination of feeling how your body moves in space.

Grounding- an approach you can use to establish an emotional and energetic boundary between you and your client and connect your energy into the earth.

Hydrotherapy- the use of water as a treatment.

Kinesthetic Experience- body awareness that one brings to life experience.

Leverage- the mechanical use of your body to apply pressure downward and forward with the least amount of muscular activity.

Massage- manual therapy involving pressure and manipulation of tissue.

Movement- an act of changing location or position of your body.

Motion- the act or process of moving or the way in which somebody or something moves.

Observation- the attentive watching of your body.

Repetitive Motion- movements that are done constantly over a period of time.

Rest- restoring and renewing the physical body after exertion.

Self-Care- focusing on the maintenance of good mental and physical health.

Vasoconstriction- narrowing of the blood vessels resulting in a contraction of the muscular wall of the vessels. The opposite of vasodilation.

Vasodilation- widening of the blood vessels resulting from relaxation of the muscular wall of the vessels. The opposite of vasodilation.

References

Anderson, Annie. www.exploreclimbing.com

Anderson, Bob. 2000. Stretching. Bolinas: Shetter Publications.

Barrett, Stephen. Sept 2003. *Surgical Pearls: Expert Insight on Peripheral Nerve Surgery For Tarsal Tunnel Surgery.* Podiatry Today. 16:9: 26-29.

Barron, Patrick. 2003. Hydrotherapy Theory and Technique, Third Edition. St James City: Pine island Publishers Inc.

Benjamin P, Tappan F. 1998. Tappan's Handbook of Healing Massage Techniques. Stamford: Simon and Schuster.

Bradford, N. 2000. Complementary Health. Great Britain: Hamlyn.

Braun M, Simonson S. 2005. Introduction to Massage Therapy. Baltimore: Lippincott Williams & Williams.

Brecher, P. 2000. Secrets of Energy Work. New York: Dorling Kindersley Publishing, Inc.

Buchman, Dian Dincin. 2002. The Complete Book of Water Healing. New York: Contemporary Books.

Byrne, Rhonda. 2006. The Secret. Hillsboro: Beyond Words Publishing.

Cash, Mel. 1996. Sport & Remedial Massage Therapy. London: Ebury Press.

Chaitow, Leon. 1995. Learning How To Assess Postural Muscles. *Child Life Essentials, Bodywork Masterclass* Series 4; www.healthy.net.

Collinge, William. 1996. Massage Therapy and Bodywork: Healing Through Touch. www.healthy.net.

Collins, Elise Marie. 2006. Chakra Tonics. San Francisco: Conari Press.

Dahong Z, Lade A, Wong J. 1998. Chinese Exercises & Massage for Health and Longevity. NY: Hartley & Marks Publishers, Inc.

Davies, Clair. 2004. The Trigger Point Therapy Workbook, Second Edition. Oakland: New Harbinger Publication, Inc.

Delisa JA. 1984. Tibial Nerve Branching at the Tarsal Tunnel. *Arch Neurol*, 41:645-646.

Dixon, Marian Wolfe. 2001. Body Mechanics and Self-Care Manual. New Jersey: Prentice Hall.

Evans, Maja. 1992. The Ultimate Hand Book. San Francisco: Laughing Duck Press.

Fritz, Sandy. 1995. Mosby's Fundamentals of Therapeutic Massage. St. Louis: Mosby-Year Book, Inc.

Frye, Barbara. 2000. Body Mechanics for Manual Therapists. Standwood: FRYETAG Publishing.

Grant, Keith. October 2003. Massage Safety: Injuries reported in Medline relating to the practice of therapeutic massage 1965-2003 . *Journal of Bodywork and Movement Therapies*. 7 (4): 207-212.

Greene, Lauriann. 1995. Save Your Hands! Seattle: Infinity Press.

Hajic, Marjorie. Hand Health resources.com

Juhan, Deane. 1998. Job's Body. Barrytown: Barrytown, Ltd.

Kome, P. 1998. Wounded Workers. Toronto: University of Toronto Press.

Lowe, W. 2006. Muscle Strains. June:6. Massagetoday.com

Little, Tias. 2001. The Ground Up. *Yoga Journal*. Nov:81.

Maran, C. 2003. Weight Training. Ontario: Thomson Course Technology.

McGinnis, Peter. Biomechanics of Sport and exercise. *The Self Coached Climber.com*

Pascarelli, Emil, Quilter, Deborah. 1994. Repetitive Strain Injury; A Computer User's Guide. John Wiley and Sons.

Payne L, Usatine R. 2002. Yoga RX. New York: Broadway Books.

Pershic G. Tarsal tunnel syndrome. Emedicine.com: Web Md.

Riggs, Art. 2002. Deep Tissue Massage. Berkley: North Atlantic Books.

Sarasohn, Lisa. 2006. The Woman's Belly Book. Norato: New World Library.

Schiffman, Eric. 1996. Yoga The Spirit and Practice of Moving Into Stillness. New York: Pocket Books.

Shelton, L. 2005. The Ultimate Body Book. Carlsbad: Hay House.

Solomon, Louise. 2003. Yogalates. New York: Sterling Publishing Co.

Svirinskaya, Alla. 2005. Energy Secrets. Carlsbad: Hay House, Inc.

Tarkan, Laurie. Athletes' Injuries Go Beyond the Physical. The New York Times: Health. Wed June 18, 2008.

Unkown author. 2007. Associated Massage &Bodywork Professionals. July. www.massagetherapy.com

Unknown Author. 1993. New England Journal of Medicine. Jan. 328:282-283.

Unknown Author. 2006. Massage Therapy Fast Facts. Associated Bodywork & Massage Professionals. July.

Upton A and McComas A. 1973. The Double Crush in Nerve Entrapment Syndromes. *Lancet.* 2:359-362.

Virtue, Doreen. 2004. Angel Medicine. Carlsbad: Hay House, Inc.

Virtue D, Lukomski J. 2005. Crystal Therapy. Carlsbad: Hay House, Inc.

Werner, Ruth. 1998. A Massage Therapist's Guide to Pathology. Baltimore: Lippincott Williams & Wilkins.

Williams, Anne. 2006. Spa Bodywork: A Guide for Massage Therapists. Baltimore: Lippincott Williams and Wilkins

Wilson, Paul. 1995. Instant Calm. New York: Penguin Group.

Wilson, Stanley. 1997. Qi Gong For Beginners. Portland: Rudra Press.

Index

194

Author/ Course Instructor

Karina Braun, BS, LMT, NCTMB is a Licensed Massage Therapist, Yoga Instructor, and Reiki Master. She had her own practice and co-owned a hair salon and spa in Texas for 5 years. Yogamotion training in 2001 benefited both herself and her clients in assuming self-care. In 2002, the instructor moved to Las Vegas, taught at a massage school, and worked at a well-known spa on the Las Vegas Strip. Karina resides in Las Vegas doing part-time massage, writing educational material, and enjoying life.

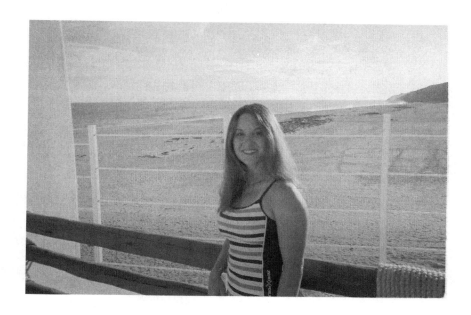

Order Form

Web orders: www.igetintouch.com
Telephone orders: 702-576-3288
Please have Visa or MasterCard ready
Postal orders:
Mail to: Get In Touch, 5546 Camino Al Norte #2-173, N Las Vegas, NV 89031

Name: _____

Address: _____

City: _____ State: _____ Zip: _____

Telephone (   ) _____

Book prices are $29.95 each
Book with Home Study Course $125.00
Each home study course includes 10 nationally approved CE hours from NCBTMB once test is completed and certificate of achievement is awarded.

Sales Tax: Please add 7.75% for books shipped to Nevada addresses.
Shipping: $8.00 for the first book and $2.00 for each additional book. Bulk order discounts are available.
International orders: Please call 702-576-3288
Number of Books_____   Number of books plus home study course_____

Subtotal_____
NV residents add 7.75% tax_____
Shipping_____
Total_____

Payment:
☐ Check   ☐ Credit Card: ☐ Visa   ☐ MasterCard
Card number: _____
Name on card: _____
Expiration date: _____
Security Code: _____
Signature_____

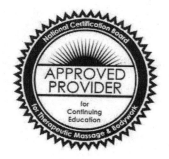

197